# exercise
## yourself
thin

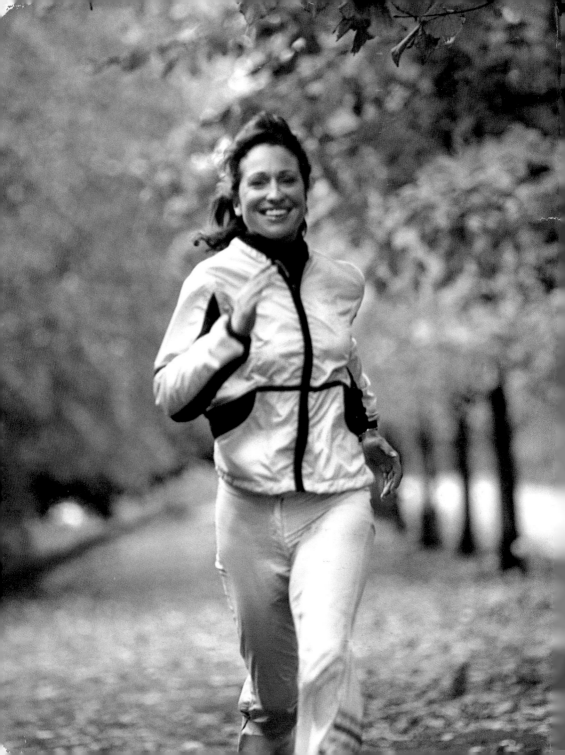

# joanna hall

YOUR
ONE-STOP
GUIDE TO A
BEAUTIFUL
BODY

# exercise
## yourself
thin

First published in Great Britain in 2008 by
Kyle Cathie Limited
122 Arlington Road, London NW1 7HP
www.kylecathie.com
The material in this book comes from Joanna Hall's *The Weight-Loss Bible*

10 9 8 7 6 5 4 3 2 1

ISBN 978-1-85626-836-3

Project editor Vicki Murrell
Designer Abby Franklin
Photographer Dan Welldon
Production Sha Huxtable

A Cataloguing In Publication record for this title is
available from the British Library.

Printed by TWP, Singapore

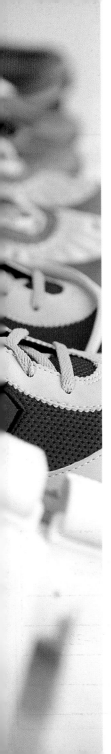

# Contents

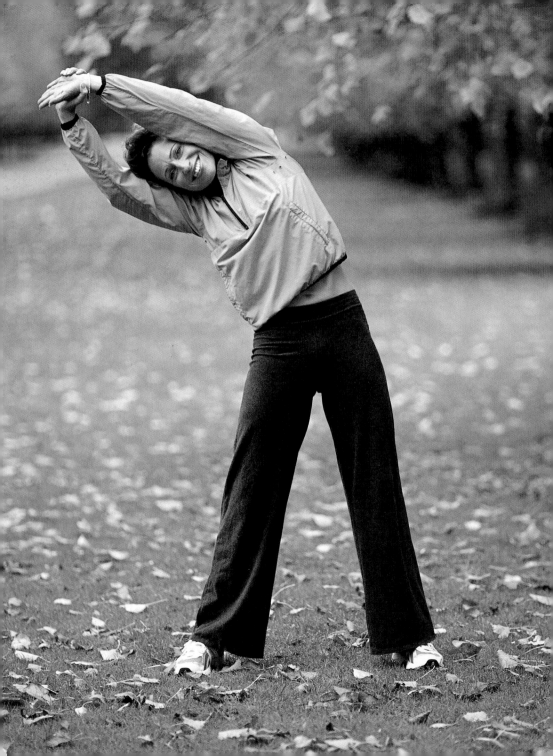

# Introduction

Exercise means different things to different people. It may mean sweat and tears on the rugby pitch, hordes of sweaty bodies pounding flesh in the gym, the lone runner crossing barren terrain, or just plain and simple walking. However, we all seem to be in agreement about one thing: we need to take exercise to become fitter and healthier. Exercise makes us feel good, improves our health, reduces our stress and slows down the ageing process – and to enjoy the benefits it does not have to be as arduous as you may think. You don't have to be able to run a half marathon to enjoy good health – total wellbeing is a combination of mind and body. If you are motivated to lose a little weight, reduce your blood pressure, or your risk of heart disease, stroke and some cancers then the best thing you can do is start being active.

One of the most important things we need to do is challenge the way we think about exercise – let's stop beating ourselves up if we don't have time to work out three times a week, and instead think about navigating each 24 hours. You'll find lots of effective plans and programmes in this book so that, even when you are struggling with your motivation, there will be a tip to focus you again and haul things back under control. And if you're just plain bored with going to the gym, have a change and maybe go for a swim or a dance class, just as you would treat yourself to a new outfit if you were fed up with all your clothes.

And remember, never ever underestimate how walking can change your body. It's the cheapest and easiest option so why not make it the foundation of your weight-loss programme and, with the right pace and technique, which you will find in chapter 2, I promise you will see results fast. So go on...

Be active
Joanna

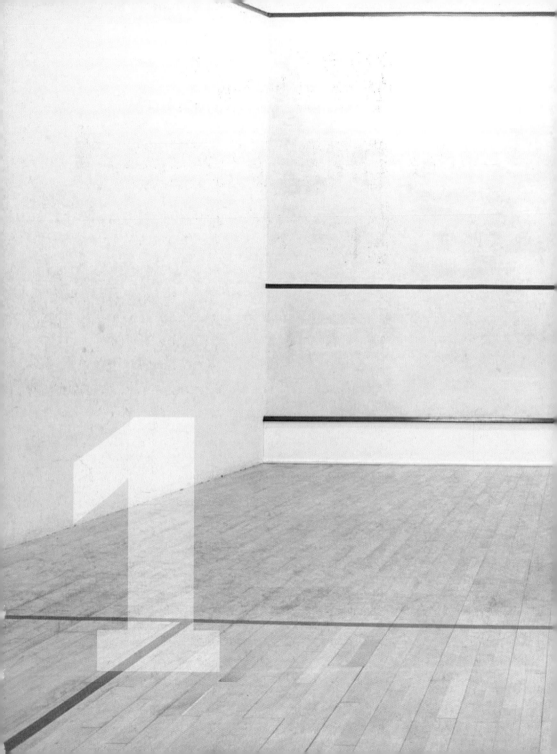

# What you need to do

# The benefits of an active lifestyle

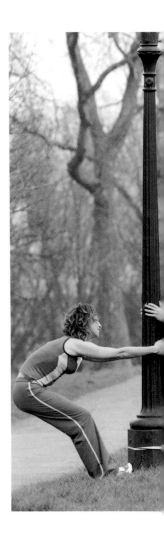

In a recent study, published in the American Journal of Clinical Nutrition, researchers looked at the energy expenditure of women who had lost weight the year before. The single distinguishing feature between those who had successfully kept their weight off and those who had regained the pounds was physical activity. Their energy expenditure was a staggering 44 per cent higher than the women who had regained weight.

Even more encouraging is the emerging evidence that moderate exercise can provide significant health benefits for people who are currently inactive. New health-related guidelines highlight the importance of 30 minutes or more of physical activity at least 3 times per week. This is the equivalent to a brisk walk of a total of 7–9km/5–6 miles for most healthy adults. Whatever your age or circumstances, exercise is a physical investment well worth making.

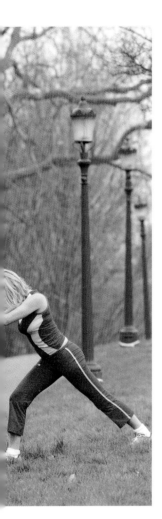

### REGULAR AEROBIC EXERCISE REDUCES BLOOD PRESSURE

Studies show that regular aerobic exercise reduces systolic and diastolic blood pressure by about 10mm Hg. A word of caution, though: if your resting blood pressure exceeds 200/105, you should not take part in an aerobic exercise session.

### EXERCISE ALLEVIATES DEPRESSION

Research suggests that exercise generally improves mood, and regular, moderate exercise can be as effective as medication and psychotherapy in combating depression. Even a 20-minute walk in woodland and open spaces can reduce stress and change brainwave frequency to the more stress-reducing alpha waves.

### SMALL BOUTS OF EXERCISE REDUCE CHOLESTEROL LEVELS

In tests, people who exercised for 3 10-minute sessions a day showed greater improvements in blood cholesterol levels than those who exercised for half an hour in a single session.

### EXERCISE PROTECTS POST-MENOPAUSAL WOMEN AGAINST DIABETES

Studies found that women between the ages of 55 and 69 who exercised regularly were 31 per cent less likely to develop diabetes than those who did not. And if you exercise moderately or vigorously more than 4 times a week, your risk of diabetes is half that of women who rarely or never exercise at these levels.

### PHYSICAL ACTIVITY REDUCES OBESITY

Regular exercise is the key to maintaining healthy body fat levels and The National Registrar of Obesity has shown successful body fat loss has been maintained in clinically obese individuals when they participate in regular physical activity that burns 4,000 calories a week.

### EXERCISE IMPROVES GLUCOSE INTOLERANCE

Regular exercise and physical activity can improve blood glucose regulation and reduce the need for diabetic medication.

# The Energy Gap

We'll start with the basic principle for weight loss – the Energy Gap. If you want to lose weight, you have to create an Energy Gap – put simply, you have to expend more calories through moving your body than you consume through food and drink. The bigger the Energy Gap, the more weight you lose. It's that simple. And if you can sustain the gap, the greater your long-term success will be.

## HOW TO CREATE AN ENERGY GAP

How you move your body I refer to as physical activity, and this broadly falls into three categories:

- Lifestyle Activity
- Occupational Activity
- Structured Exercise

In this chapter, you will see that much of the most effective physical activity for long-term weight management isn't difficult or vigorous, but it does need to be done consistently.

## HOW YOUR BODY USES ENERGY

Your body is constantly expending energy in different ways.
- The energy we need to function – for breathing, or for keeping our hearts beating, for example – is referred to as Resting Metabolic Rate (RMR).
- The energy we use to process our food – the digesting, absorbing, metabolising and storing of nutrients – is called the Thermic Effect of Food.
- And the energy we use as we move around – be it Structured Exercise, Occupational Activity and Lifestyle Activity – is called the Thermic Effect of Exercise.
These three energy forms add up to total energy expenditure. Discovering how each one relates to your overall energy expenditure will help you create your Energy Gap.

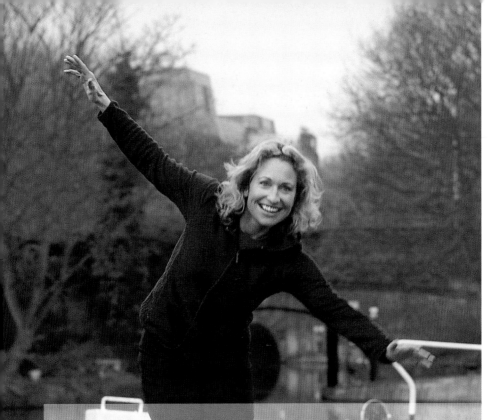

## HOW THEY COMPARE?

Your Resting Metabolic Rate has the greatest potential impact on your total energy expenditure, accounting for 65 to 75 per cent of the energy your body burns. Your RMR is strongly linked to the amount of muscle mass you have. A pound of muscle will burn between 50 and 60 calories a day, whilst a pound of fat burns fewer than 10. Surprisingly, very low calorie diets (less than 1,100 to 1,200 kcal per day for women, 1,400 to 1,500 kcal per day for men) have been associated with a reduction in RMR. This reduction can actually encourage your body to store fat rather than burn it – not what you want to happen.

The Thermic Effect of Food requires approximately 10 per cent of the energy consumed at any one sitting, and is the smallest contributor to total energy expenditure.

The Thermic Effect of Exercise is the most variable component of total energy expenditure, as it depends on your level of daily activity. Absolutely anyone can increase their total energy expenditure – whether you like to stick on your training shoes or not.

# How active do you think you are?

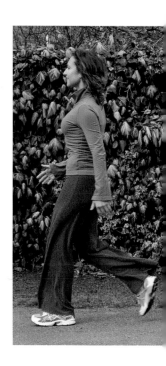

Ask someone if they have an active life, and they'll most probably tell you how busy their day has been. But think about it. Okay, so you may feel tired in the evening, but is it because you were mentally, geographically or physically active? Here's what I mean. You take the kids to school, finish off a report, get the washing done, take a parcel to the post office, pick up a prescription from the doctor, do half a day at the office, pick up the kids at 4pm, take Johnny to football, Elizabeth to piano, cook the dinner and do some homework for your evening class. By the end of the day you are tired because you have had a mentally exacting day, having to juggle and complete so many tasks, and because you have been geographically active, covering a great many miles – but mostly in a car or bus. In fact, you have barely moved at all.

## HOW ACTIVE ARE YOU REALLY?

An effective way of finding out is by filling in a 24-hour Activity Chart. This chart allows you to record your level of activity by simply colouring each hour according to what you are doing during that time. Once it's completed, you can put your day into perspective and see at a glance how often you are actually physically active. You'll also be able to see when you may be able to squeeze in a little more activity. If one day tends to be quite different from the next, you can extend your chart to cover a few days, or perhaps even a whole week. This will give you a fairly good visual indication of how much you move your body over a period of time. Remember, it is the consistency of your actions that reaps the rewards on your weight-loss journey.

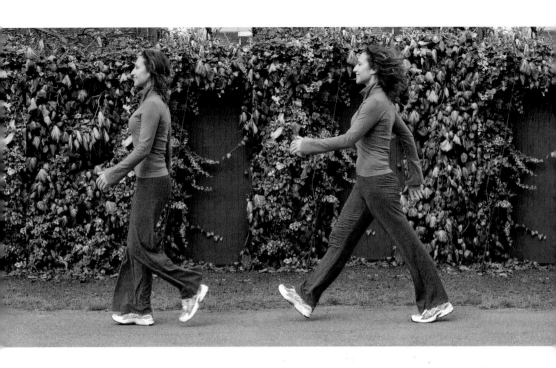

## 24-HOUR ACTIVITY CHART

| 24 | 1 | 2 | 3 | 4 | 5 | 6 | 7 | 8 | 9 | 10 | 11 | 12 | 13 | 14 | 15 | 16 | 17 | 18 | 19 | 20 | 21 | 22 | 23 |
|----|---|---|---|---|---|---|---|---|---|----|----|----|----|----|----|----|----|----|----|----|----|----|----|

**Think of your typical day as you colour in this chart**

- Colour in black the time you are lying down
(sleeping, napping or stretched out on the sofa).
- Colour in pink all the time you are sitting
(at work, in a vehicle, at home; include such things as watching TV, reading, at a desk or computer, eating, and all sedentary leisure activities).
- Colour in orange the time you are on your feet (doing light activities in your day).
- Colour in yellow the time you are doing strength or resistance work
(include heavy manual lifting).
- Colour in green the time you are doing moderately intense physical activity
(such as brisk walking).
- Colour in purple the time you are doing vigorous physical activity

# How much do I have to do?

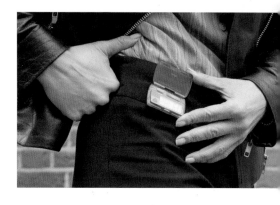

Between 45 and 90 minutes of moderate-intensity physical activity per day will prevent unhealthy weight gain and keep you within normal BMI range. Sixty minutes is the average recommendation, and should prevent you becoming overweight, or becoming obese if you are already overweight (source: the International Association for the Study of Obesity). This 60-minute recommendation is equivalent to a calorie burn of approximately 300 kcal for someone weighing 75kg (165lb) (this is on top of your RMR).

Please bear in mind that 60 minutes is the average recommendation; it's possible that you may need to be aiming for closer to 90 minutes, depending upon your starting-point, your goals and your personal metabolism. So don't feel daunted; you can do this.

## HOW CAN I MEASURE MY ACTIVITY LEVELS?

A good way of finding out how active you are is by wearing some sort of tracking device. The simplest and easiest of these is a pedometer. At the end of each day you can record the number of steps you have accumulated on your 24-hour colour chart (see page 15). If you don't want to use a pedometer then you can make a note of how much time you spend walking each day. The trouble with this, however, is that it's not very accurate – studies have shown that we tend to overestimate how physically active we are by a whopping 51 per cent!

## WHAT IS A PEDOMETER?

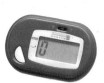

A great tool, and to my mind an essential item in your weight-loss tool kit, a pedometer records the number of steps you take a day. It works by measuring the up-and-down motion of your hip as you walk. It will also measure movements you perform during your day, in addition to walking, such as climbing the stairs, gardening or getting in and out of your car. I'd strongly encourage you to invest in a reliable one. If you wear my Big Steps pedometer correctly, it has 99 per cent accuracy and, in independent research, was shown to be the most accurate when walking at different speeds on different terrains (for more info, see page 111).

Here's how to wear it. Slide the clip onto your belt or waistband. The most common position is directly above and in line with your knee, but you may have to experiment to find the best place for your shape. If your tummy protrudes over your waistband or belt, it may cause the pedometer to tilt and not work properly. If this is the case try wearing it more to the side of your body.

### Count your 10,000 steps

Ideally you should aim to achieve 10,000 steps a day (roughly equivalent to a distance of 8km/5 miles). But don't panic if you are not quite there yet; slowly increase your current number of steps by 5–10 per cent each day. If you walk 5,000 steps one day, aim to increase this to between 5,250 and 5,500 the next. Also remember that any improvement at all will get you going in the right direction. Monitor your progress and you'll feel confident in the knowledge that you are doing what you need to do to widen your Energy Gap and see a change in your body. This will all foster a winning relationship between your body and your brain and set you on the road to success.

### Why 10,000?

▪ Studies have shown that taking 10,000 steps a day without any dietary adjustment can prevent any weight increase, although it may not cause weight loss on its own.

▪ It also provides a fail-safe foundation for your physical activity and exercise – when life gets busy, the first thing that tends to go is Structured Exercise; by maintaining your 10,000 steps, however, you're still achieving your basic calorie burn.

▪ Walking is beneficial to your overall health, reducing your risk of developing serious illnesses such as heart disease, some cancers, diabetes and depression. It is also a load-bearing exercise that helps to prevent osteoporosis.

▪ The 10,000 steps message encourages you not to sit down for too long; if you get up and move every 30 minutes throughout the day, you'll soon clock up those steps.

## HOW DO YOU RATE?

Once you have filled in your 24-hour Activity Chart and established your average number of steps per day, have a look at the table below, drawn up from research conducted in Japan as a means of classifying activity levels.

| Under 5,000 steps a day | 'sedentary' |
|---|---|
| 5,000–7,500 steps a day | 'low active' |
| 7,500–10,000 steps a day | 'somewhat active' |
| 10,000–12,500 steps a day | 'active' |
| 12,500 steps a day + | 'highly active' |

# Lifestyle and Occupational Activity

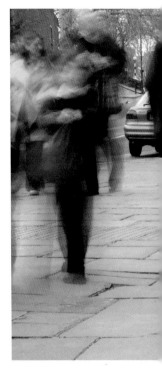

As we know, Structured Exercise plays a major role in our overall energy expenditure, but it's not the only way to burn off calories. Your body expends energy every time it moves, so your day-to-day activities, whether at work (Occupational Activity) or in your own time (Lifestyle Activity), all contribute to weight loss.

According to a report published in the International Journal of Obesity, people who consistently took short bouts of physical activity ended up expending more calories than those who took longer bouts of Structured Exercise. Remember: your fat cells will not be able to differentiate between a machine at the gym and a flight of stairs at work. The more you move your body, and the more energetically you move it, the greater amount of energy your body will burn and the more weight it will lose.

## HOW CAN I DO IT?

Remember: all calories count, independent of the intensity of the activity. If you reduce the time you spend on sedentary things like watching TV, you will free up time for more active pursuits. Small changes such as this, systematically incorporated into your lifestyle, can help widen your Energy Gap. In practical terms, you can achieve your target by accumulating more steps throughout your day as well as taking more vigorous Structured Exercise. Here are a couple of ways to help you achieve this, which I've called 'Active Travel' and 'The Workout Wedge'.

## ACTIVE TRAVEL

Here are the keys to active travel:

### In the workplace

- Stop wearing your mobile phone like a part of your body! Leave it where you will have to get up to answer it.
- When possible, avoid emailing colleagues in the building – get up and talk to them. An American study recently reported that using email for 5 minutes out of every hour in your working day could result in a kilo of weight gain every two years – that's potentially 5kg (11lb) of surplus fat by 2016!
- Walk down as well as up the stairs.

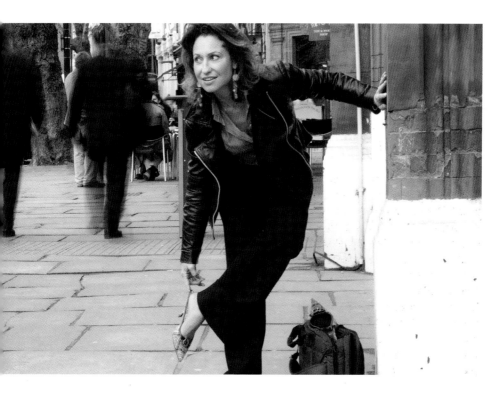

Apart from accumulating more steps, it's better for you: the impact your body absorbs can help safeguard against osteoporosis.

- Do a chore at lunchtime. Everyone has errands. Be savvy and get something done that involves you moving. Post that letter, pay that cheque in at the bank.
- Piggy-back a habit. Find something you do each day – whether it is buying the newspapers, reading your post or having your morning coffee – and aim to put an additional 1,000 steps on your pedometer before you do it.

**At home**

- Banish all remote control devices for a week. If you want to change channels or put another CD on, get up and do it!
- If you've got a cordless phone, keep moving while you talk.
- Play interval games with the kids! On walks, take it in turns with your partner or friend to push the buggy while the other one runs races with the older children; then swap over to catch your breath.
- One last thought... Whether at work or at home, use the loo on another floor. The average person goes to the loo five times a day, so you'll be climbing and descending an extra flight of stairs every day.

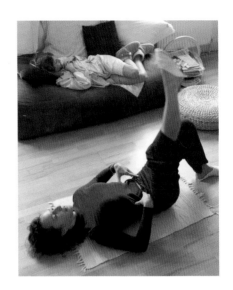

# Navigating the 24

My concept of Navigating the 24 is all about increasing your overall physical activity levels through each and every day, encouraging you to move more, more often, wherever you are. The times when you can be more physically active do add up when you start thinking about it.

**Consider this:** there are 24 hours in the day and 7 days in the week. That makes 168 hours in each week. Let's say we have the luxury of getting 10 hours' sleep each night (unlikely, I know – 10 just keeps the arithmetic simple, and maths was never a strong point of mine!). This leaves us (168 – 70 =) 98 hours when we are awake and have the potential to be physically active. Let's suppose we take an hour's structured exercise three times a week, as this is the amount we are generally advised to take and probably the maximum most people think they can squeeze into a busy life. This leaves us with (98 – 3 =) 95 hours when we can move our bodies.

Have a look at the table opposite and you will soon see how easy this can be. On an average day, the less active person burns just 30 per cent of the calories the active person uses. If they compensate by going to the gym, they will still use only 60 per cent of the calories burnt by the active person (who does not go to the gym). In addition, the active person keeps their metabolism revved up right through the day. This means they burn an extra 2 calories a minute – which may not sound much, but add that up over 24 hours, 7 days a week, 12 months a year and you soon notch up an extra million calories! That's why you should always opt for the active alternative.

| Less active person | kcals | |
|---|---|---|
| Get someone else to iron while you sit down | 34 | |
| Get someone else to vacuum while you sit down | 11 | |
| Prepare pre-sliced vegetables | 3 | |
| Microwave a ready meal | 3 | |
| Drive children a half-mile to school | 11 | |
| Drive three miles to work | 24 | |
| Use lift to travel up four floors | 1 | |
| Chat with colleagues for 20 minutes at lunchtime | 26 | |
| Shop by internet | 17 | |
| Watch TV for two hours | 175 | |
| Mow the lawn with power mower for 10 minutes | 50 | |
| Read a newspaper for half an hour | 34 | |
| **Basic total** | **389** | |
| Compensatory gym workout (60 minutes) | 403 | |
| **Revised total** | **792** | |

| Active person | kcals | difference |
|---|---|---|
| Iron for 30 minutes | 77 | 43 |
| Vacuum for 10 minutes | 40 | 29 |
| Wash, slice and chop your own vegetables | 28 | 25 |
| Cook for 30 minutes | 67 | 64 |
| Walk children a half-mile to school | 56 | 45 |
| Cycle three miles to work | 135 | 111 |
| Climb four flights of stairs | 11 | 10 |
| Walk and chat for 20 minutes at lunchtime | 78 | 52 |
| Walk a mile to the shops and back | 311 | 294 |
| Take a brisk one-hour walk | 336 | 161 |
| Use a hand mower for 10 minutes | 68 | 18 |
| Play with children for half an hour | 94 | 60 |
| **Basic total** | **1301** | **912** |
| No gym workout | 0 | -403 |
| **Revised total** | **1301** | **509** |

(Energy expenditure for a 63.5kg/10 stone person.

Source: British Heart Foundation health promotion unit, University of Oxford)

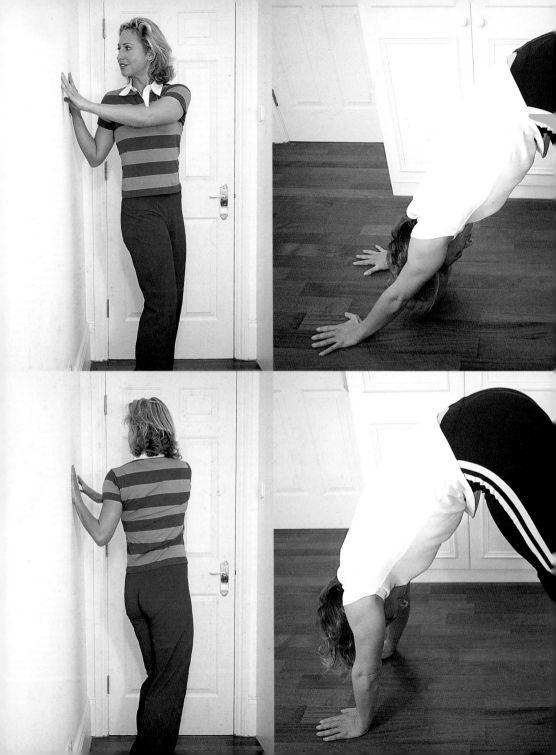

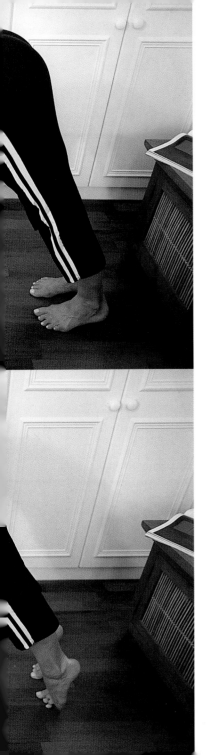

# The Workout Wedge

The idea behind this is that you wedge a workout in between other activities in your day. A Workout Wedge should be at least 2 minutes long, and there's no end to how inventive you can be with it. Here are a couple of ideas.

■ Look back at your 24-hour Activity Chart (on page 15) and see where you may be able to wedge in a workout – on your way to work, when you get back home in the evening, in your lunchtime, while the bath is running, or the computer is downloading some software... with a little thought you can be quite creative.

■ Try the dinner workout wedge! A number of my clients found this effective, since it targets that time of day when resolve is weak. You get home, you're starving, you're tired, and you can't be bothered to exercise. Wedging in a workout while your dinner is cooking is beneficial in several ways: completing exercise before you eat actually helps you eat less, and leaves you feeling more energised. It really is as simple as prep, exercise and eat! Many dishes take about 20–25 minutes to cook once the preparation's done – and in that time you could...
– Follow a 20-minute exercise video...
– Jog round the block a couple of times...
– Do some stretches, climb some stairs... or try some exercises, such as the Waistband Whittler workout on pages 52–53. It's quick and easy to do!

## BAD WEEK? NOT NECESSARILY...

Many people who are trying to lose weight perceive a 'good week' as one when they've got to the gym three times, and a 'bad' week as when they've only managed to attend once or perhaps not at all. (A recent survey revealed the average gym member only shows up once a week!) In fact, if you've been quite physically active in your work and leisure time you may have expended quite a bit of energy without realising it, and have not had a 'bad' week at all.

Try to recognise every small achievement, as our success tends to carry over into other behaviour patterns, so it seems easier to make better food choices or decrease portion size. And, of course, the opposite is also true.

Ideally, a 'good week' will include Structured Exercise as well as Occupational and Lifestyle Activity, as you navigate your way through each 24 hours. So even though this should encourage you to be much more physically active throughout your day, taking time out to do some structured exercise is still important. Exercise intensity improves your fitness and maximises your calorie burn. In addition, you will soon start to experience other benefits, such as increased energy. You'll also sleep better and feel great! This is not just a pleasant side-effect: feeling good about yourself is a vital part of your weight-loss journey. Let's take the next step now.

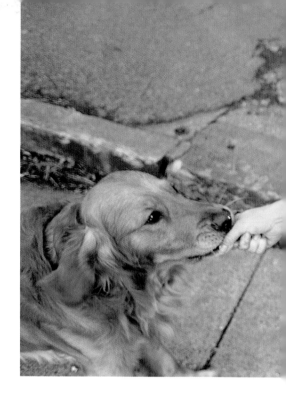

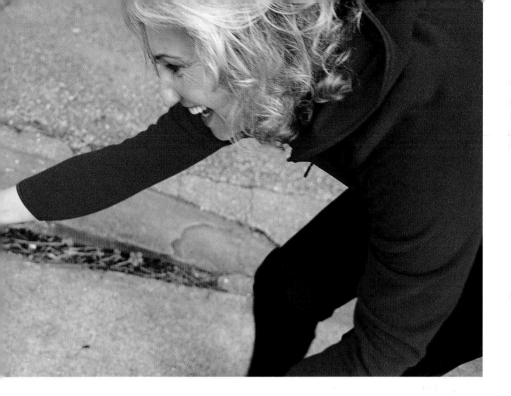

## WHAT DO YOU WANT TO ACHIEVE?

Now is the time to give a little more thought to what you would personally like to achieve. You need to be quite specific about this. All the workouts and tips in this book will help you become fitter, healthier and feel better about yourself, but what is it that you really want to get out of this book? Just as you may set goals for yourself in your professional life, so you may wish to set yourself some realistic physical targets. Once you have decided what these are, this book will help you achieve them, building your physical confidence and changing how you feel about yourself. Maybe you have your summer holiday to work towards and want to feel confident in your swimsuit. Maybe there is a local charity run you would like to take part in. Perhaps your doctor has told you that you need to exercise to reduce your blood pressure, or maybe you want to learn to relax and sleep better. If you are concerned about the health and fitness of those around you, you'll find exercise workouts for the whole family, including the kids. And what you want to achieve today may be different in 6 months' time, a year on from now, or maybe when you reach the next decade. Regular exercise will help you have lots of energy and a good outlook, whatever your age, and this book will be your companion as you go through life, to help you be fit, be healthy, be your best shape and most of all BE ACTIVE!

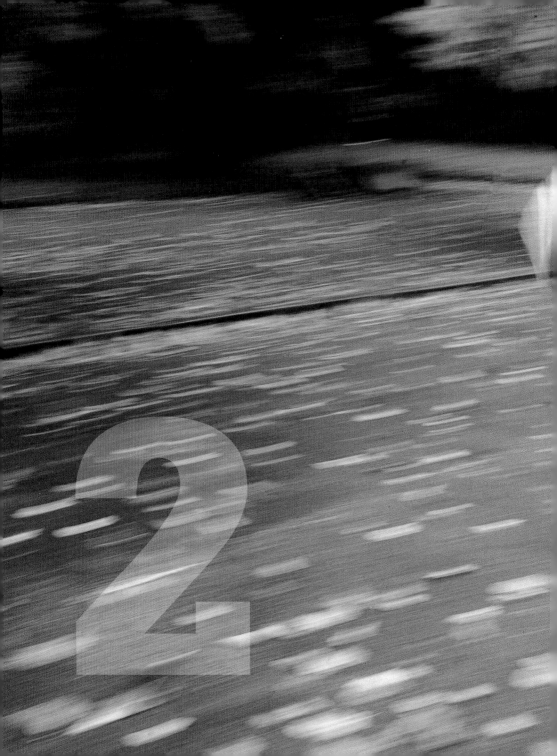

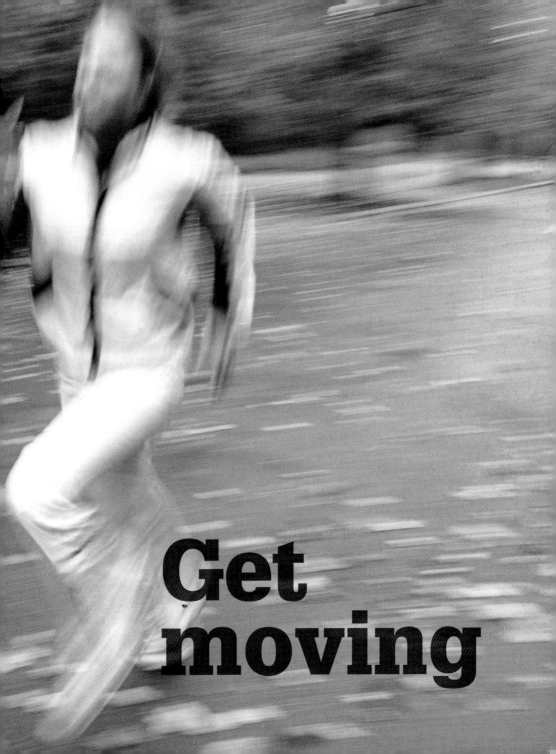

# Get moving

# Structured Exercise

So far, we've seen how moving your body can create that all-important Energy Gap – and we've looked at ways in which you can incorporate physical activity into your daily life. With Structured Exercise, however, you have the power to really blast that fat. Basically, the harder you work and the longer you are able to sustain that effort, the more calories you will burn. But don't panic if you are not a natural lover of exercise – there are lots of things to try that don't involve going to the gym. Remember: variety will keep you motivated, and just because you don't like one sort of exercise, it doesn't mean to say that you'll never find anything you enjoy. Ideally, Structured Exercise should combine cardiovascular, resistance and flexibility routines.

## CARDIOVASCULAR EXERCISE

This is often termed 'endurance' or 'aerobic' (as the large muscles of the body it targets require lots of oxygen to move). It is a good all-round calorie-burner and is usually the most effective method of expending energy in an exercise session.

**Cardiovascular exercise should:**
- use the large muscles of the body in a continuous, rhythmic fashion;
- be relatively easy to maintain at various workout intensities;
- be enjoyable.

A useful way to optimise energy expenditure in endurance exercise is to vary the intensity. You can do this with forms of exercise that can be easily adjusted or graded to overload the cardio-respiratory system (for instance, increasing the grade of a treadmill or pedalling resistance during stationary cycling). If you're walking or running outdoors, you can increase your pace, and seek out some hills. It's not hard to build periods of intensity into your exercise plans.

## RESISTANCE EXERCISE

This causes your muscles to contract to lift a weight. It could be your own body weight, equipment in the gym or even a household object – it doesn't matter, as long as your muscles are made to contract to overcome a force. Resistance exercise tones muscles, and it helps maintain your muscle mass, which can start to decline from your late 20s, so it will make a useful contribution to your long-term weight management.

**Building muscle**
The main function of resistance exercise in weight loss is to build muscle tissue – one of the most metabolically active kinds of tissue in the body. The more muscle you have, the higher your Resting Metabolic Rate – the calories needed at rest to

maintain all of the body's vital processes and systems. The largest component of the body's total calorie expenditure is the energy needed to maintain its RMR, therefore increasing RMR helps to burn more calories. One study showed a 7 per cent increase in RMR in people aged 56–80 after they completed 12 weeks of resistance training.

## FLEXIBILITY ROUTINES

These involve stretching and moving your joints. Although they tend to be less physically demanding and therefore burn fewer calories, they can be really enjoyable and also figure as important components of a warm-up and cool-down. Flexibility work such as yoga and Pilates often proves to be a good introduction to Structured Exercise, especially if you feel you are not a natural exerciser, and the very idea of getting hot and sweaty fills you with inertia!

## CAUTION

Exercise affects many different body systems. Muscles need a greater supply of energy, so the heart and lungs work faster and more efficiently to keep them well supplied with oxygenated blood. Blood vessels in the intestines, liver, stomach and kidneys narrow so that more blood is directed away from these areas and to the muscles. Regular exercise helps to reduce blood pressure and prevent the build-up of fatty deposits in the arteries, relieves the symptoms of peripheral vascular disease, increases bone density and muscle mass and can help to relieve depression. However, if you have any of the following conditions, you should check with your doctor or specialist before starting an exercise programme.

- If you haven't exercised for some time, or are obese on the BMI scale, consult your GP or a fitness instructor. A walking programme would be a good starting point for you.
- If you have coronary heart disease or a history of heart problems, your doctor may refer you for an electrocardiogram (ECG) before you embark on an aerobic exercise programme. This will usually involve you walking, running on a treadmill or cycling an exercise bike while your heart rate is monitored, to see how well you cope with the increased stress.
- If you have had a fracture, dislocation or cartilage injury over the last few years, it is worth seeking advice from a physical therapist or osteopath about the types of exercise that won't put stress on the area in question.
- Anyone with a chronic condition like asthma, osteoarthritis, osteoporosis, high blood pressure or diabetes should follow their GP's advice on the exercise that will be best for them.

In all cases, respect your body. Always start out gradually and don't overdo it. If something hurts, or makes you feel dizzy or short of breath, just stop and seek advice.

# What kit do I need?

You don't have to spend a fortune on exercise kit and special equipment, but there are a few items that can make the whole exercise experience a lot more enjoyable. You might want to consider the following:

- **A cap with a peak** – keeps both rain and low sunlight off your face and out of your eyes.
- **A warm hat** – You can lose up to 60 per cent of your body heat through your head, so in winter a warm hat can be a smart investment. It will also keep long hair under control on a windy day, but make sure it won't blow off.
- **Gloves** – In cold weather your extremities can get pretty chilly. Invest in a pair of gloves with some grip so you can wear them on a bike or while pushing a buggy. Many sports varieties are made using breathable, comfortable and functional materials – find them at sports shops.

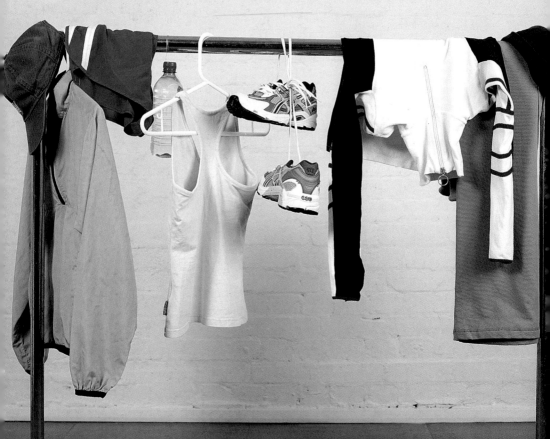

- **A lightweight waterproof** – important to keep you dry in spring showers or autumn downpours. For convenience, get one that can roll up quite small.
- **Heavier waterproofs** – good for the wettest weather. I actually use golf waterproofs and have found them to be both functional and attractive.
- **Breatheable tops** – a long-sleeved one for cooler weather and a sleeveless one or a T-shirt for when it's warmer.
- **Legwear** – invest in something with some stretch – there are many stylish leggings available. Shorter legwear – calf, knee or thigh length – is more comfortable in warm weather. Ultimately go for whatever you feel most comfortable in.
- **Cycling shorts** – buy these if you are intending to do quite a bit of cycling – personally, I think they are worth it.
- **Sunglasses** – Yes, you can still exercise with style. Even when it's not that bright, wearing clear lenses will keep grit and pollution out of your eyes.

## TRAINERS:

Shoes are crucial. You don't have to spend a fortune, but getting a good, well-fitting pair is money well spent. Be aware that an old shoe may look in good condition when its supportive qualities have diminished considerably with wear. When buying trainers, bear the following in mind:

- Shop for shoes in the afternoon, because feet tend to swell during the day.
- Athletic shoes should be comfortable from the start, requiring minimal breaking-in.
- When trying on shoes, try them out on both carpet and hard surfaces, simulating an outdoor walking or running experience in the shop.
- Before you part with your cash, run through this checklist: FIT, COMFORT, CUSHIONING and CONTROL. Don't buy trainers, no matter how much you like the look of them, unless they provide all four of these qualities.
- Replace your athletic shoes every 300 to 500 miles (or 4–6 months). Your feet may carry you as far as 12,000 miles in your lifetime – so take care of them.

### REMEMBER THIS:

**Cushioning** – protects the foot from injury
**Flexibility** – transmits the power of your body efficiently
**Stability** – controls the motion of the foot and ankle (so you don't get sprains, strains or even fractures).

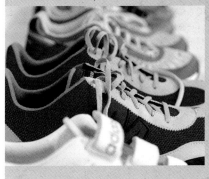

# How hard
# do I have to work?

With Lifestyle and Occupational Exercise, consistency is the key but with Structured Exercise it's how hard you are working that truly counts as it's here that you can develop your fitness and build up the amount of energy you burn. But what is most important is working at the right intensity for your safety, enjoyment and success and therefore I strongly advise monitoring of some sort:

## HOW TO MONITOR INTENSITY

Some methods are simpler than others, but it's vital to choose at least one. Exercising too hard will not be enjoyable, and will increase your likelihood of giving up as well as your risk of injury; not exercising hard enough will not yield results.

## HEART-RATE MONITORING

Heart rate increases in proportion to exercise intensity, so recording heart rate is a fairly accurate measure. Heart-rate monitoring can be done manually, or by using a piece of equipment such as a heart-rate monitor watch. Most heart-rate monitors give you an immediate reading, and some models even allow you to set training limits.

To monitor your heart rate manually, you can record your pulse either at your wrist or at your carotid artery. This can be found at the side of the neck; extend your chin away from your shoulders and, with your first and second finger, apply a small amount of pressure on either side of your windpipe. You should feel a small pulse underneath your fingers.

A heart-rate training zone is between 50 and 85 per cent of your maximum heart rate. If you are new to exercising, you should start off at the lower end of this range and gradually work upwards. To calculate, use the following equation:

**For men: 220 minus age**
**For women: 228 minus age**

From here, you can work out your own specific training zone by calculating 50 and 85 per cent of your personal maximum heart rate.

**For example, if you are a 35-year-old woman: 228 – 35 = 193 (personal maximum heart rate)**
**50% of that (193 x .50 = 96.5)**
**85% of that (193 x .85 = 164)**

Please note that as your cardiovascular fitness improves, your heart rate response will be lower for the same absolute exercise intensity. This means that you will have to work at a higher intensity to achieve the same energy burn in the same amount of time.

If all these calculations seem a little daunting, don't fret – there's a much simpler way, described in the chart opposite, which many of my clients prefer:

| Rating | Perceived Exertion | Examples of Exertion | Clothing/Sweat Factor | Chat Factor |
|---|---|---|---|---|
| 0 | Nothing at all | Lying completely still in bed, sleeping | Warm clothes or covers required as body is still and not generating heat. No sweat. | Can sleep-talk to your heart's content! |
| 1 | Very, very weak | Watching TV or a film in the cinema, sitting in a boring meeting at work, sewing, or reading a book. | Layer of clothes dependent on temperature of environment. No sweat. | Can chat to your heart's content |
| 2 | Weak | Browsing in the shops, playing the piano, typing on your laptop, eating dinner, sitting and chatting with friends, filling dishwasher. | Layer of clothes dependent on temperature of environment. No sweat. | Can chat to your heart's content |
| 3 | Moderate | Walking the dog, walking to work, playing a leisurely game of doubles tennis. | Feel a little warm in the clothes you are wearing. Starting to sweat. | Able to talk comfortably |
| 4 | Somewhat strong | Climbing escalators, carrying the shopping up several flights of stairs, cycling for pleasure. | Feel like you need to take off an item of clothing and tie it around your waist. Starting to perspire on your body and face. | Able to talk but not sing. |
| 5 | Stronger | Manually mowing your lawn, walking very briskly. | Need to take off a layer of clothes to avoid sweating. | Able to hold a breathy conversation. |
| 6 | Harder | Walking briskly up a hill, or walking very very fast, pushing a pram up a slope, digging in the garden, lightly jogging. | Perspiration felt on body and face. | Able to hold a conversation but it's something of a struggle… uncomfortable. |
| 7 | Strong | Fast jogging or running, lifting heavy objects such as furniture or weights in the gym. Can only continue for a limited time. | Appropriate clothing worn to allow body to breathe. Definite sweating on face and body. | Able to hold a sporadic conversation with short pauses for breath |
| 8 | Very Strong | Running fast to catch the last bus home, skipping with a rope, circuit training. Have to force yourself. | Body feeling very warm. Sweating. Light clothing worn to allow movement. | Unable to hold a continual conversation (you're mostly monosyllabic). |
| 9 | Very, very hard | Running in a race. | Body feels very hot. Sweating during and immediately after activity. | Unable to hold a conversation. |
| 10 | Maximum effort. You can work no harder. | Running for your life. | Your whole body and head feel very hot. | Unable to speak. |

# Getting fitter on your weight loss journey

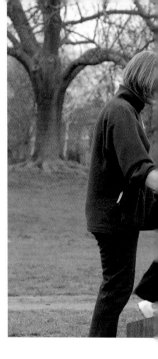

As you get fitter, you will find that the exercises you started with become easier.

- Make your Structured Exercise sessions longer
- Gradually increase your exercise intensity in small increments. Boosting your effort by 5–10 per cent is a good way to progress.
- Exercising using different of pieces of equipment in a gym can be challenging, as different muscle groups are involved.
- Introduce interval training.

## INTERVAL TRAINING

Interval training combines periods of high-intensity work with moderate- to light-intensity work. It is highly effective, and can be a useful form of exercise to complement an active lifestyle, helping you improve your fitness as well as aid weight management. Design your interval-training programme according to how fit you are, how long you plan to exercise and what your specific aims are. You are the one in control: you select the form of exercise you wish to do, you apply the intensity and you are away. Here is a sample interval-training programme, intended to enhance the body's calorie-burning capacity.

**Always start gradually** with a 3–5 minute warm-up of light-intensity cardiovascular exercise to prepare the lungs, heart and muscles for the workout to follow. Try steady walking, rolling the shoulders and circling the arms.

**Train for 4 minutes** at a high intensity followed by 4 minutes at a moderate to light intensity. Try brisk walking interspersed with more moderate walking.

**Alternate** these 4-minute intervals for the entire workout. During the high-intensity interval, you should feel 'comfortably challenged' (a PRE of 7–8). During the moderate-intensity interval you should feel 'somewhat challenged' (a PRE of 5–6).

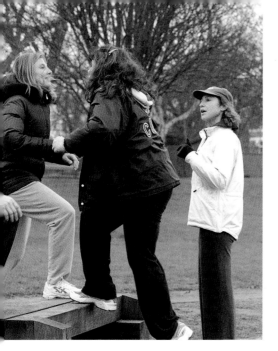

**Start off** with a 20-minute workout and gradually progress up to 60 minutes over several weeks. Your rate of progress will depend on your fitness.

To get fitter and keep burning calories you need to exercise to a point of 'overload'. This is when your body feels physically challenged. As long as you can hear your body saying to you 'Oh, that feels a bit harder – what's going on here?', you can be sure that you have provided 'overload'.

## MEASURING YOUR FITNESS PROGRESS

Just as you're keeping track of the changes in your body shape and weight, it's also useful – and very gratifying – to see how fit you're becoming. There's a

variety of ways to do this, but one of the simplest and easiest is with a timed walk of a set distance. It could be a kilometre or a mile, or a favourite route, but it has to be somewhere you can return regularly without a problem. Note down your heart rate when you start, when you finish, and then again a minute later, as well as the time it takes to complete your route. As you get fitter, your heart muscle becomes stronger and is able to pump the oxygenated blood your body requires more efficiently. Over a period of time, you should expect to see not only a faster walking time but a drop in your heart rate as well. Try to test your fitness every four weeks.

### Start heart rate
This is your resting heart rate, taken immediately before your walk. Find your pulse (either wrist or neck will do), record your HR for 10 seconds and multiply it by six.

### Finish heart rate
This is your heart rate immediately after your walk. Find your pulse and record your HR for a full 60 seconds (it will start to slow down during this time).

### Recovery heart rate
After you have recorded your finish HR, wait one minute and then record your HR for a further 60 seconds. This will give you the greatest indication of how your fitness has improved over the 28 days. The faster your heart returns to its normal rate the more efficient it is.

# Injury prevention

As you become increasingly active, you may come up against a few niggling aches and pains in various parts of your body. This is to be expected if you are new to exercise, particularly if you have begun to walk a lot more. Many of these can be easily minimised with a little know-how. Try these tips, which will even help you burn more energy at the same time.

## AVOID SHIN PAIN

**Foot roll:** Standing with your feet almost together, roll up onto your toes, hold for 2 seconds and roll back down. Then roll onto the outside of your feet, hold for 2 seconds and roll back down. Next roll onto your heels with the toes off the ground, hold for 2 seconds and roll back down. Repeat this sequence 10 times before every walk.

## AVOID KNEE PAIN

**Straight leg raise:** Sit on the ground with your legs extended in front of you. Bend your right leg and place your right foot flat on the ground. Rest your hands behind you and sit up straight. With your left foot flexed, contract your left thigh and raise your leg 15–30cm (6–12 inches) off the floor. Hold for 5 seconds and then lower. Do 10 lifts, and then switch sides. Perform the sequence 2–4 times a week.

## AVOID ACHING LEGS

**Hip and calf stretch:** Stand with your feet together, then step your right foot about 3–4 foot lengths in front of you. Both feet should be pointing forward. Bend your right knee so it is just above but not in front of your right foot. Check both big toes are facing forward. Keep your left leg straight and your left heel on the ground to feel a stretch in your left calf. Flatten your lower back and tuck in your pelvis so you also feel a stretch in the front of your hip. Hold for 4–7 slow deep breaths, release, and repeat on the other side. Stretch each leg twice after each walk.

**Lower calf stretch:** Stand close to a tree and rest the ball of your right foot on the trunk so that your heel is still on the ground. Bend your right knee in towards the post; you should feel a stretch in the lower part of the calf. Hold for 10–15 seconds and repeat twice each side. Do this at the end of each walk.

## AVOID UPPER ARM TENSION

**Upper body stretch:** Stand with your feet about shoulder-distance apart and raise your right arm over your head, bending your elbow so your right hand is behind your head. Place your left hand on your right elbow and gently pull your elbow to the left, allowing your upper body to bend slightly to the left. Hold for 4–7 deep breaths, release and repeat on the other side. Stretch each side twice after every walk.

# TIPS FOR TOP TECHNIQUE

How you perform your exercises will not only affect your rate of progress but also your risk of injury. The following simple tips will help you build a fit, strong body and achieve better results in less time:

**The mistake:** Rolling the knee inwards so it is not aligned with the toes when you are performing lunges, step aerobics or pliés. This can injure the knees.
**Put it right:** Keep knee and toes in line. Make sure as you look down you can see your toes. Imagine drawing a line down the front of your knee cap – if you extend it all the way down, it should be in line with your second toe.

**The mistake:** Leading with the chin in abdominal exercises in an effort to curl the upper body off the floor. This puts strain on the neck and lessens the effectiveness of the exercise, because you are using your neck and shoulder muscles instead of your abdominals.
**Put it right:** Lift from the breast bone. Imagine the movement starts from the breast bone. Keep the chin and neck in line by imagining that your ear lobes and collarbone are always in alignment.

**The mistake:** The walking stomp! As you increase your walking speed, technique can be compromised and the foot tends to land heavily rather than in a controlled way.
**Put it right:** Keep your upper body lifted as you walk, imagining you have a cup of water balanced on each shoulder that you mustn't spill. Focus on walking through the whole foot as you land as well.

**The mistake:** Slumping as you step up. Often when you step up onto a bench or even the stairs your body remains slumped and the legs, back and hips never fully extend. This puts pressure on your spine, hinders posture and may contribute to injury.
**Put it right:** Make sure you extend upwards fully each time you take a step. Keep your head high and be proud of the space your body occupies.

# Choose your cardio exercises

So… you've done your homework and you've learned a lot. Now it's time to have fun. You'll soon see from the list on the following pages that cardiovascular exercise is not all about treadmills and stationary cycling!

The world is your oyster! You can opt for intrepid sports like whitewater rafting or Himalayan climbing, or activities that fit in with your lifestyle, such as skipping with your children in the back garden or cycling to work. The following list includes some obvious and some less common suggestions, with advice on how to perform them and what they will do for you (as well as the calories you can burn).

## WALKING

**What you do:** Walking is the simplest, most accessible and least expensive form of exercise, and it works for the vast majority of people. To make walking an effective form of structured exercise, however, you need to establish your optimum walking pace.

First of all, get yourself somewhere where there is plenty of room. Start walking and gradually pick up your speed – swinging your arms faster will help. Continue to increase your pace until you feel yourself involuntarily breaking into a jog. This is known as your break point. From this point, drop back to your walking pace, and you now have your optimum walking pace. You should feel like you are walking with a purpose, and much faster than you normally would.

Here are a few postural hints for perfecting your technique:
- Strike the ground with the heel first, rolling through the foot then pushing off with the toe.
- Think 'tall' – don't slump into your hips.
- Pull in your abdominal muscles to support your back.
- Relax your shoulders and let your arms swing naturally without crossing your body.
- Use your natural stride – don't try to lengthen it. If you want to increase your pace, try moving your arms faster – your legs will naturally speed up.
- Wear properly cushioned trainers that fit you snugly but without pinching.

**Great for:** As well as burning calories, it streamlines your hips and thighs.

**How much you burn:** Up to 180 calories in 30 minute

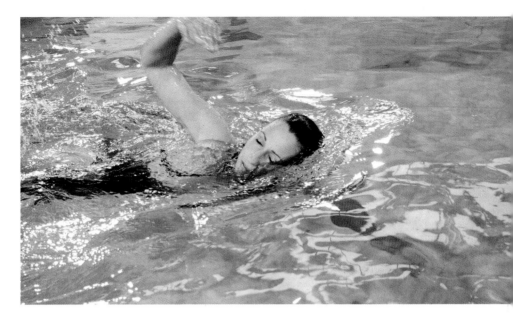

## BELLY-DANCING

**What you do:** When you think belly-dancing, you may think Middle-Eastern restaurants. Don't. There are now any number of classes around the country providing tuition in more cultured styles. Egyptian belly-dancing is more classical and skilful, while the Turkish style tends to be more overtly sexy!

**Great for:** Boosting your self-esteem in a non-competitive environment, getting your heart bumping and increasing your body awareness – as well as teaching you a few extra little moves to show off on the dance floor or the bedroom! The waist and midriff will become more toned and shapely, and you should also find you get better mobility in your spine.

**How much you burn:** Up to 140 calories in 30 minutes.

## SWIMMING

**What you do:** Since the water provides a certain degree of support, energy expenditure can be quite low but get competent at swimming and you can make swimming part of your regular aerobic exercise together with more weight-supporting workouts. Aqua classes can be fun and also provide toning benefits due to the resistance of the water.

**Great for:** Swimming involves the whole body and is fantastic if you suffer from joint problems as the water can provide support to limbs especially if you're arthritic.

**How much you burn:** Up to 190 calories in 30 minutes.

## SALSA AEROBICS

**What you do:** A South American dance brought into the studio. It's just what you need if you want to exercise but don't want to feel like you're working out.

**Great for:** Strengthening your heart and your lungs. Targets the often-neglected oblique muscles that help trim and define your waist.

**How much you burn:** Up to 150 calories in 30 minutes.

## BODYJAM

**What you do:** Bodyjam incorporates a variety of dance techniques that are simple and easy to follow.

**Great for:** Developing a sense of achievement as you master dance routines while your heart and lungs get a good cardiovascular workout at the same time. It'll also tone your thighs and bottom, and the arm movements will help with your overall co-ordination.

**How much you burn:** Up to 180 calories in 30 minutes.

## ICESKATING

**What you do:** Grab some friends and head down to the local ice rink. It's great fun!

**Great for:** Your balance – and once the basic moves are mastered, you'll benefit from a firmer bottom, streamlined legs, greater poise and better posture. You'll also get a great workout just from getting up every time you fall over!

**How much you burn:** Up to 234 calories in 30 minutes.

## JOGGING

**What you do:** Either indoors on a treadmill or outdoors in the fresh air, jogging or running is an excellent all-round aerobic exercise. Make sure you have good supportive shoes and when starting out alternate brisk walking with jogging. Try 30 seconds' jogging to 60 seconds' walking and gradually reduce the ratio of walking to jogging until you can jog continuously for 20 minutes.

**Great for:** Improving the stamina of your heart and lungs. It's a good energy burner as you are having to support the whole of your body as you move.

**How much you burn:** Up to 300 calories in 30 minutes.

## TENNIS

**What you do:** Tennis as a calorie burner can be a little deceptive. Vigorous energetic games of tennis can be great fun and a wonderful excuse to get outside, but do be aware that the stop-start nature of the game and the social nature of this great sport can mean you burn fewer calories than you might think.

**Great for:** Toning arms and legs, as well as a cardio workout if you run for those wide balls.

**How much you burn:** depends on intensity of game.

## THAI BOXING

**What you do:** A form of martial arts using bare hands. Lessons are widely available in gyms and martial arts centres. It originated in medieval times when arms, legs, elbows and knees were all used as weapons in close fighting. Nowadays the ancient spiritual connections are still maintained and are embedded in the rules of the sport.

**Great for:** Building strength through agility and cardio fitness. It is a great form of self-defence as well being good for boosting confidence and self-esteem.

## BALL SPORTS

**What you do:** Whether it's basketball, netball, rounders or football, ball sports are great fun and you don't always need to put together a team to enjoy messing around with a ball.

**Great for:** Hand-eye co-ordination and cardio fitness. The social element of these activities can be a great motivator to keep you exercising so combine them with healthy picnics in the park on Sundays and get a whole group of you playing.

**How much you burn:** depends on the sport and your position in the team (for example, goalkeepers won't burn so many calories as midfielders).

## ROCK-CLIMBING

**What you do:** Many large leisure centres and outdoor pursuits centres have specially designed climbing walls. If you want to be at one with nature, specialist courses can take you to stunning locations such as the Dolomites

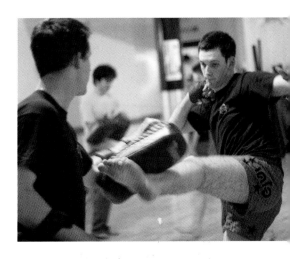

in Italy, the Brecon Beacons in Wales, or the Cairngorms in Scotland.

**Great for:** All-round muscle strength and tone. The step-up action is especially good for toning buttocks and thighs and the whole body co-ordination challenges mind and body.

**How much you burn:** depends how challenging the climb is.

## CIRCUS TRAINING

**What you do:** There are a number of circus schools and courses up and down the country. Some holiday companies now offer circus skills classes as part of their activities programme. If you have ever been to a circus and thought 'I would love to try that' – then here's your chance.

**Great for:** Improving overall body awareness, self-esteem and body confidence. Dependent on the circus skills you choose, you can improve your upper and or lower body, tone and improve agility and flexibility.

## CYCLING

**What you do:** Use your bike to run errands, or cycle to school with the kids – it's a fantastic way for exercise to creep into your day. You'll be surprised how on shorter journeys you can often get to your chosen destination quicker than by car.

**Great for:** All-round cardiovascular exercise that's especially great if you've got children. Since body weight is supported, and the pressure applied to the pedal is relative to the weight of the cyclist, both adults and children can cycle together quite easily, without the child feeling exhausted before Mum and Dad! Follow cycle routes around places of interest or discover great pubs out in the country. If you're mountain biking your thighs, arms and upper back will gain definition, while more level cycling can be a significant calorie burner.

**How much you burn:** Up to 240 calories in 30 minutes.

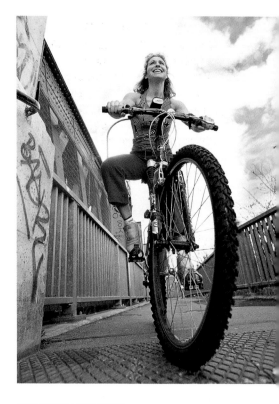

## GOLF

**What you do:** Walk the golf course and you will be clocking up significant steps on your pedometer.

**Great for:** The rotational nature of the golf swing can be great for a toned torso but do start out slowly – remember the Tiger Woods and Nick Faldos of this world spend hours training to help create a balanced smooth swing.

**How much you burn:** Up to 130 calories in 30 minutes.

## HORSE-RIDING

**What you do:** The horse may appear to be doing all the hard work – but in reality you're getting a good lower-body toning session, plus a healthy dose of fresh air. It is less cardiovascular than other activities, however.

**Great for:** Calming you, and stimulating the release of feel-good brain waves. Your inner thighs and lower abdominal muscles benefit from horse-riding, and you have to focus on having good posture to ensure you stay on your horse!

**How much you burn:** Up to 120 calories in 30 minutes.

## DOWNHILL SKIING

**What you do:** Swoosh down the slopes, preferably on skis, not your backside is totally exhilarating, and enough to give any fitness cynic a massive adrenaline high.

**Great for:** Working the legs and abdominal muscles. Using your poles to help you get up small inclines will target your arms, too.

**How much you burn:** A cool 374 calories an hour.

## SNOWBOARDING

**What you do:** It's akin to surfing on snow, as you stand sideways on a board. Snowboard teachers claim a novice of any age can be gliding down slopes competently within a few days. You never know – you may even be overtaking the kids!

**Great for:** Your legs and buttocks; it also tones your waist and abdominals.

**How much you burn:** This full-body blast burns about 400 calories an hour.

## SNOWSHOEING

**What you do:** Snowshoeing is just walking in the snow but with special footwear. It is fast becoming the latest fashionable alpine sport, and many resorts have specially marked out scenic routes for enthusiasts.

**Great for:** Giving your thighs and buttocks a great workout.

**How much you burn:** With snow as your natural resistance, even walking at a moderate pace on flat terrain can burn as many as 500 calories an hour – more than either skiing or snowboarding will do.

## KITE-FLYING

**What you do:** Getting outdoors in pursuit of the most simple and innocent of childhood pastimes can be great fun. Take it in turns with your partner to run after the kite, collect it and set it up for its next flight.

**Great for:** Blowing away the cobwebs if you have been stuck indoors all week (remember: daylight raises your levels of Vitamin D). Boost your cardiovascular and calorie-burning efforts by finding yourself a hill, and taking it in turns to run up and down it to fetch the kite. Your hips, thighs and bottom will all benefit.

**How much you burn:** Up to 135 calories in 30 minutes.

## SKIPPING

**What you do:** Skip either by jumping with feet together (harder) or with a running motion (easier and less jarring on joints). This is intense – start with 20-second bouts and build up to 5 minutes' continuous skipping. Check that as you land your heels come down and your knees are soft.

**Great for:** Increasing the stamina of your heart and lungs. A fantastic energy burner.

**How much you burn:** Up to 280 calories in 30 minutes.

# Resistance and flexibility exercises

These can often be a useful entry point into more structured exercise sessions, since they require less physical effort. As with cardio, there's a huge range you can choose from. Here's just a small selection.

## PILATES

Pilates involves deep muscle training according to the principles of German fitness instructor Joseph Pilates. Pilates helps you to develop a strong 'core', consisting of the deep abdominal muscles along with the muscles closest to the spine, thus protecting the spine and keeping the pelvis correctly aligned. In classes, you will be shown matwork exercises that you can perform yourself, at home, and reformer exercises that need to be performed on a piece of studio equipment called a reformer (see opposite). Pilates can be good for creating a toned and sleek body without bulk, and an excellent form of exercise for improving your posture and helping to correct muscle alignment, but it has little cardiovascular value.

## YOGA

Broadly speaking, there are three styles of yoga – Astanga, Hatha and Iyengar. They differ in many ways, one of which is how much they demand of you physically. For best toning effects, opt for Astanga (or Vinyasa, which is not so well known). This incorporates more postures that are supported by body weight, and you often move from one posture to another by supporting part of your weight with your arms. Iyengar and Hatha styles are usually more gentle, and while breathing techniques are an integral part of all yoga practice, you tend to find there is more emphasis on breathing and relaxation in these two styles.

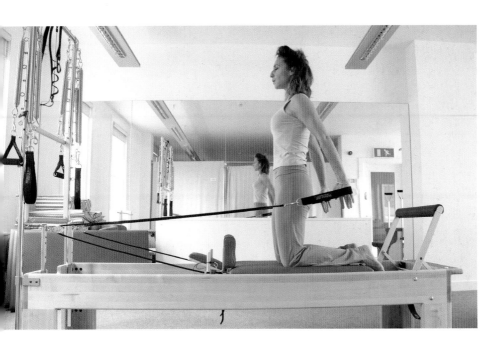

## WEIGHT TRAINING

Weight training involves the use of hand-held weights or weight machines to strengthen specific muscle groups of the body (the vast majority of health clubs will have weight-training facilities). Following a progressive weight-training programme can enhance muscle mass – but it can also make you heavier. Don't worry, however – muscle weighs more than fat, and providing you are mindful of your diet as well as your exercise regime, you will feel your clothes getting loser as your size decreases. Use weight training to complement your cardiovascular exercise, creating tone and shape in your body as you shed the fat. This means lifting lighter weights but with more repetitions, thus enhancing the

cardiovascular benefits of the workout. In the Action Plans in Chapter 5, you'll see how I incorporate resistance training to augment your cardiovascular gains and increase your energy expenditure.

## TONING CLASSES

These classes focus on resistance exercises that use your own body weight, small weights, resistance bands or balls to tone your body. Their focus will vary from class to class, but generally the idea is to increase tone with more repetitions and lighter weights.

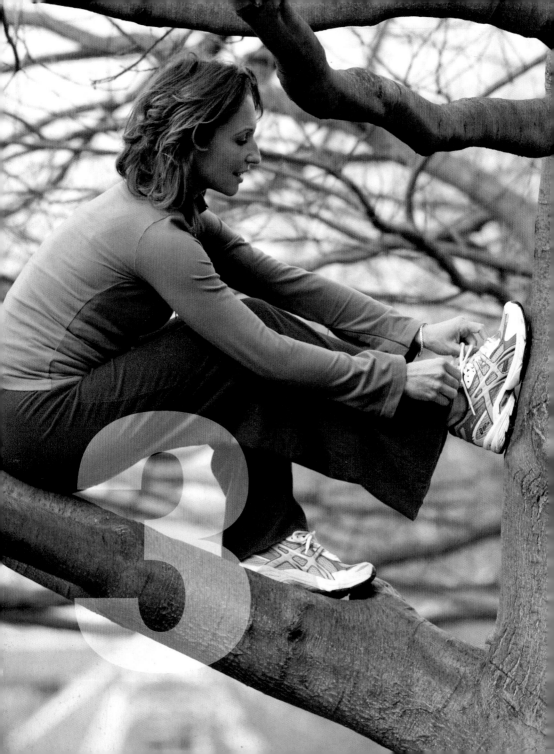

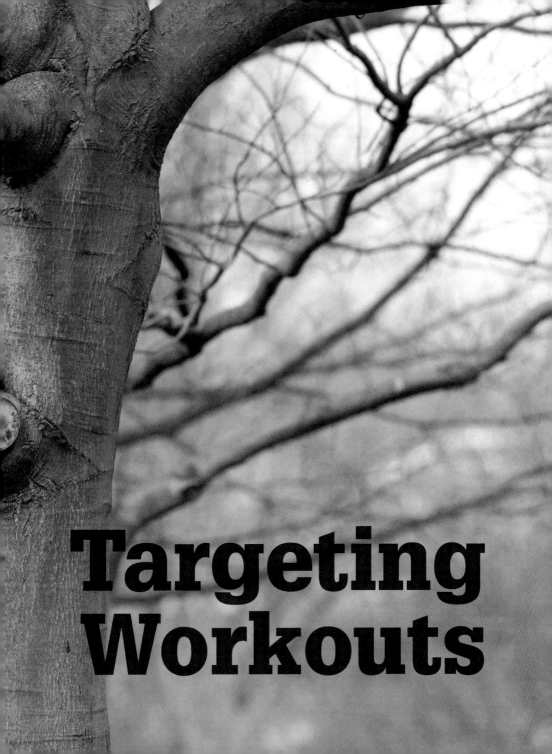

# Targeting Workouts

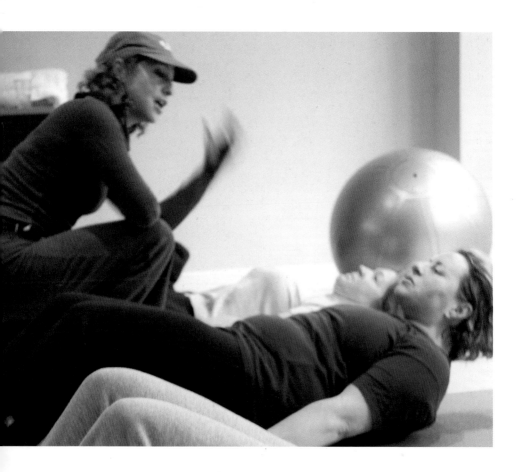

# Targeted Toning

We all have parts of our body that pose particular problems and seem to be immune to all our weight-loss efforts. This is where these Targeting Workouts come in. You can do them on your own, or use a couple of your favourite exercises as Workout Wedges or as intervals in your cardiovascular routines. First of all, let's spend a little time looking at technique, since if it's flat abs you want, it's not quantity but quality that counts. These simple flat tummy skills will help you to get great results in no time.

# THE RIB-HIP CONNECTION

**What it does:** Gives you an instant smaller, trimmer waistline.

Lie on the floor with your knees bent and place your hands around your rib cage, fingertips facing in towards your breast bone. As you take a deep breath in, feel your rib cage expand. This is how most people start their tummy exercises. STOP!! By doing this you will get a bigger waist!

To combat this, as you breathe out imagine you are wearing a corset that needs to be tightened up. As you pull your stomach down you will have engaged your internal oblique muscles, which will help you regain a 'pinched-in' waist. Try to feel relaxed and comfortable in this position.

Another method to try is to place your thumb on your lower ribs and your little finger on the top of your hip bone and draw these two points together with a small contraction of the abdominal muscles. Your spine should be in a neutral position, with a small space between the floor and your lower back. This neutral position will vary from person to person, dependent upon the shape of your spine.

Engage the rib-hip connection and neutral spine before doing any abdominal exercise.

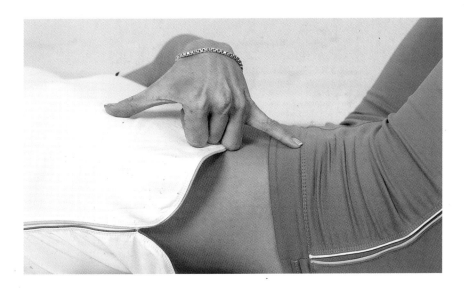

# LIFT AND LENGTHEN

**What it does:** Gives you lean, flat abdominals.

**1** Lie on the floor with your knees bent and with the rib-hip connection engaged. Start to SLOWLY lift your upper body off the floor leading with the breastbone (not the head, chin or nose).

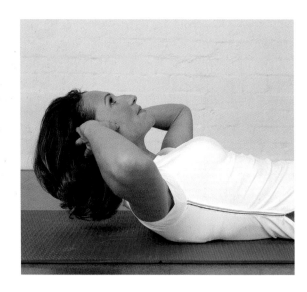

**2** Lengthen through the crown of the head as you lift and then lower again. To help you, imagine your head has to touch the edge of a semi-circle throughout the whole movement. The movement should feel long, as you lift up and down.

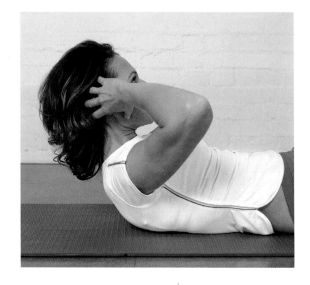

## STABLE JELLY BELLY

**What it does:** Stops troublesome lower tummy bulges and supports your back, preventing back pain.

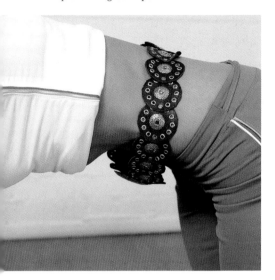

**1** To really flatten that lower jelly belly, you need to target the deep transverse abdominal muscle (the one you are contracting when you lie on the floor to do up your jeans). To help you do this, kneel on all fours and pull your belly button up to the spine and towards the ceiling as far as possible. Test how good you are at this by getting a friend or the kids to try to push your tummy a little – it should feel stable and shouldn't move.

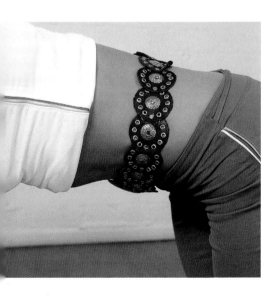

**2** Now repeat, with your tummy muscles relaxed; when someone pushes you this time, you'll notice that you wobble and have no stability.

# Waistband Whittler

The first of our Targeting Workouts, for toning those abs.

## BREAST BONE LIFT

**What it does:** Trims the upper waist and tummy area.

**1** Lie on the floor face up, knees slightly bent and feet on the floor but far enough away from your bottom so that you feel as if your toes are just about to lift up. Place your hands at the side of your head and raise your head slightly off the floor. This is your start position.

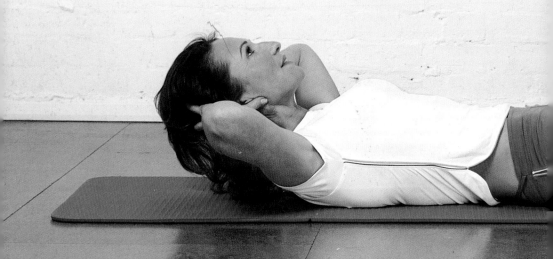

**2** From here, lift no more than 5cm, leading from the breast bone. Hold this small lift for 4 counts and lower back to the start position. Lower your head to the floor.

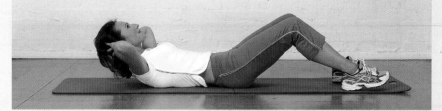

**3** **To make it harder:** start with one leg extended while the other remains bent and repeat the breast bone lift. Hold for 4 counts, then lower and repeat with the other leg extended.

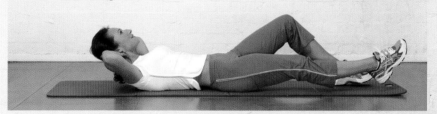

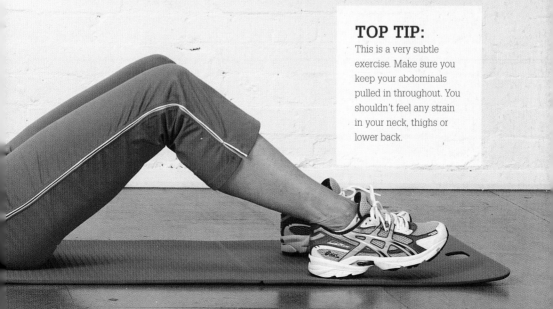

## TOP TIP:

This is a very subtle exercise. Make sure you keep your abdominals pulled in throughout. You shouldn't feel any strain in your neck, thighs or lower back.

## DEAD BUG

**What it does:** A great total tummy toner without any neck pain.

**1  Start position:**  Lie on your back and lift your legs and arms off the floor, so that your knees are bent just above your hips and your arms are directly over your shoulders, palms facing forwards. Keeping as still as possible, firmly pull your abdominals back into your spine. Hold this position for 2 sets of 8 counts.

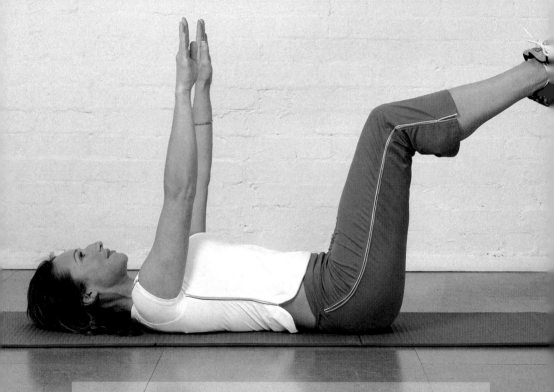

## TOP TIP:
Make sure your legs are not too close in to your body, otherwise this becomes too easy. Experiment holding your knees a little further away so you feel some tension in your abdominals.

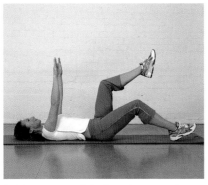

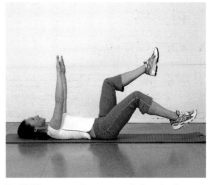

**2** Lower your right foot down to the floor and tap with your heel 4 times, without letting your lower back arch.

**3** Still contracting your abdominals, raise the right foot back up then lower your left foot to tap your heel on the floor.

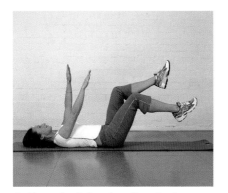

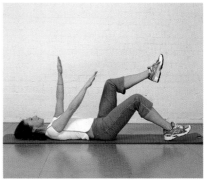

**4 To make it harder:** Start in the dead bug position. Slowly lower the right leg and right arm towards the floor at the same time. The distance between arm and knee should stay the same – imagine you're holding a beach ball between them.

**5** Gently 'kiss' the floor with your heel then slowly lift the arm and leg back up to the dead bug position. Repeat with the left arm and the left leg, keeping your abdominals firmly pulled down throughout.

## BELT PULLS

**What it does:** Flattens and improves the postural support of your abdominals.

**1  Start position:** First put on a belt that will buckle up snugly around your waist. Kneel on all fours with your hands under your shoulders and your knees under your hips. Start with your abdominals relaxed and, keeping your back straight, firmly draw in your abdominal muscles so you create space between your tummy and your belt. You should be able to slip your fingers in between your belt and your tummy. Hold this position for 30 seconds, breathing smoothly throughout. Relax for 10 seconds. Repeat 5 times.

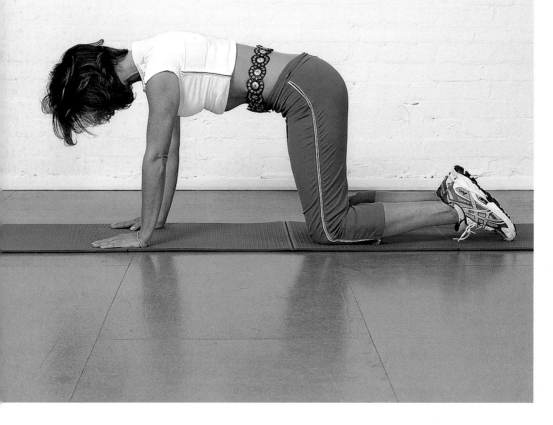

**2  To make it harder:** Keep your back straight as you extend your left arm and right leg. Now draw in your abdominal muscles firmly to create the space between your belt and your tummy. Repeat with the right arm and left leg.

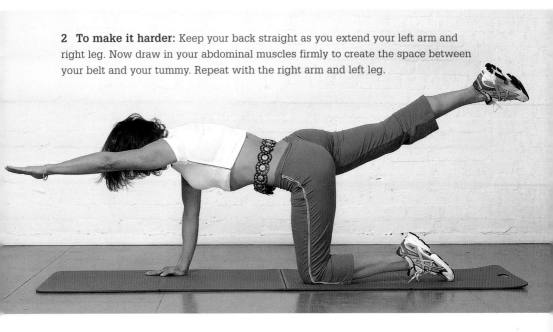

**3**  Draw your right elbow and left knee together so that they just touch. Hold for 4 counts, then extend out again. Repeat 3 times, and then draw your left elbow and right knee together and repeat 3 times.

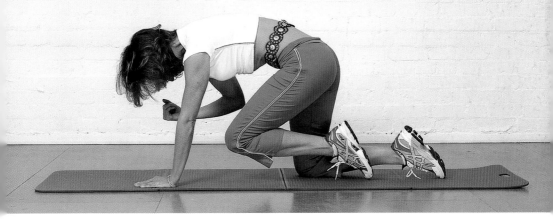

# AB REACH

**What it does:** Firms and flattens the whole of the abdominal area.

**1  Start position:** Lie on your back with your knees slightly bent and your feet positioned so that your toes are raised a little off the floor. Lift your upper body, leading from your breast bone, and place your hands on your thighs.

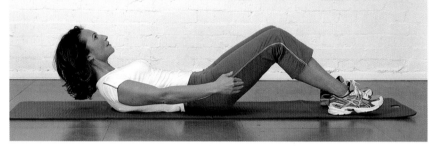

**2**  Lift about 5cm from the breast bone, trying to reach further down your thighs with your hands if you can, then lower back to your start position and extend your arms above your head, keeping your shoulders off the floor.

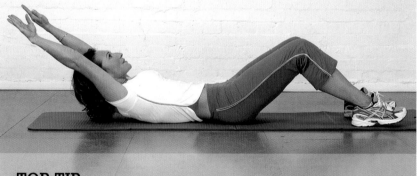

## TOP TIP:

Positioning your feet slightly further away from your bottom ensures that your spine is kept long along the floor, helping to engage and target the troublesome lower tummy area.

# OBLIQUE RIB-TO-HIP LIFT

**What it does:** Targets the waist.

**1 Start Position:** Lie on your back with your knees bent and feet extended away from your bottom. Stretch your right arm out to the side, and touch the fingers of your left hand to the side of your head. Lift your upper body from the ground.

**2** Pull your stomach to the floor and stretch across as if you are trying to fold your left shoulder towards your right hip bone. Repeat 8 times, then do the same in the opposite direction, lifting your right shoulder towards your left hip bone.

## TIPS TO PREVENT NECK PAIN

When the abdominal muscles are not strong enough to support the weight of your torso as you lift, discomfort in the neck can result. This discomfort should lessen as your abdominal muscles get stronger and firmer, so do stick with your Waistband Whittler exercises. In the meantime, however, here are a few tips to minimise neck strain.

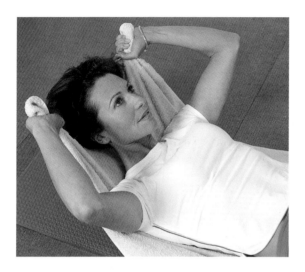

**Solution one:** Place a towel underneath your shoulders and hold onto the corners, pulling tight to cradle your head and neck as you lift. Avoid yanking your head up with your hands as you lift. Remember: always lift from your breast bone and not from your chin.

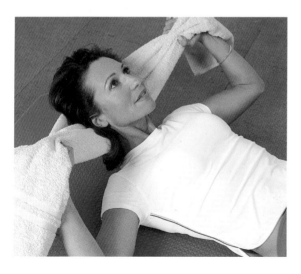

**Solution two:** Place a rolled towel at the nape of your neck and hold tightly at both ends as you lift and lower Also, strange as it sounds, press your tongue firmly against the roof of your mouth as you lift and lower. This appears to stabilise the neck muscles, giving support to your head.

# LOWER TUMMY MUSCLES 'POPPING OUT'

Sometimes as we lift, the lower abdominal muscles can 'pop' out, making the lower back unstable. Here are a couple of solutions to help train the abdominal wall to flatten.

**Solution one:** Check you have the rib-hip connection (see page 49) then place a ruler across your lower abdominal muscles. As you lift, try to keep the ruler in place by focusing on drawing down through the lower abdominal wall.

**Solution two:** Wear a belt for your abdominal exercises. Buckle it so you have room for a little movement between your abdominals and the belt. As you lift, focus on keeping your abdominals away from the belt buckle and not pressing against it.

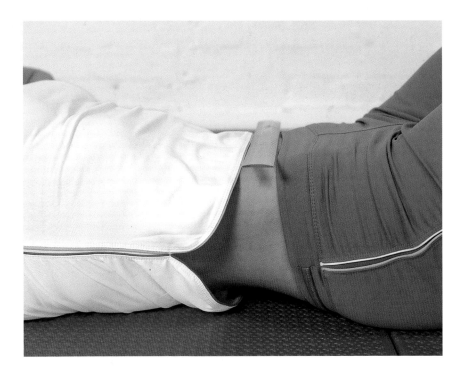

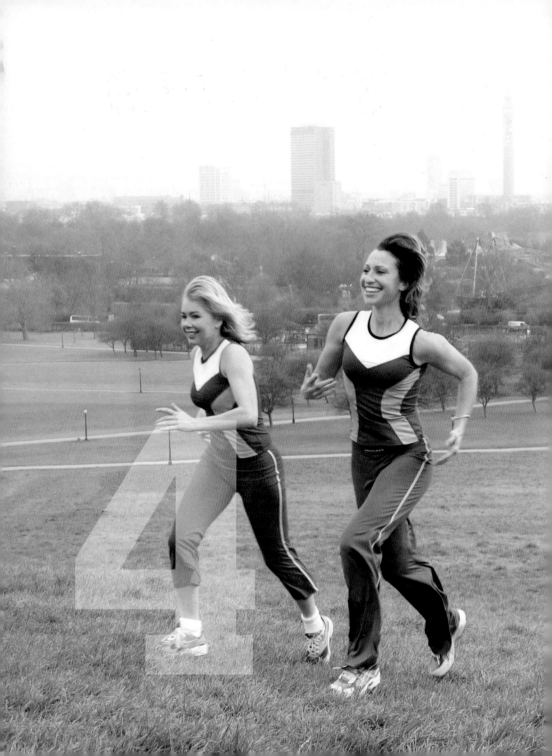

# exercises for
# specific body shapes

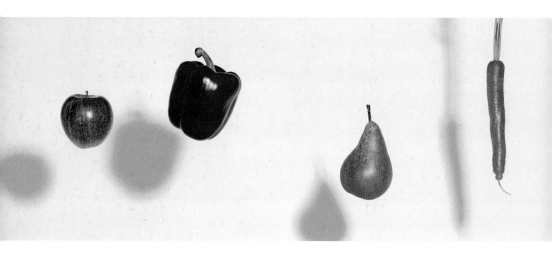

# Body shape

We have become so used to seeing incredible celebrity body transformations on television and in magazines that we seem to expect the same level of transformation from our own body. In reality, however, most of us don't have the sort of money it takes – or the luxury of air-brushing. It is possible to improve our figures but exactly how much can we change the body shape Mother Nature dealt us?

Our fundamental body shape – skeletal frame, muscle, body fat and distribution of certain hormones – is determined by our genes. According to geneticist Claude Bouchaud, our genes and the hormones we produce during puberty can determine our body shape by as much as 70 per cent... so that leaves about 30 per cent that can be redefined, moulded and determined by exercise and what we eat.

As we get older our bodies naturally lose muscle, but muscle tone can be improved and muscle size can be increased with appropriate exercise. Body fat is directly determined by energy balance – consuming too many calories and not expending them increases body fat, while expending more calories than are consumed encourages body fat reduction. But unless we undergo significant cosmetic surgery, which is a very bad idea, our basic body shape – whether we're 'big-boned' or 'petite' – is pretty fixed.

We generally fall into four broad body shapes. I've categorised them as: pear, red pepper, carrot and apple.

## WHAT SHAPE ARE YOU?

**You are more pear if:**
- your hips are wider than your shoulders
- you have a smaller upper body frame
- your top half is 1 to 2 dress sizes smaller than your lower half.

**You are more red pepper if:**
- you have an ample bottom and bust with a defined waist
- you are a classic hourglass shape
- you are prone to gaining weight and storing body fat on arms and legs.

**You are more carrot if:**
- you have broadish shoulders with slimmer hips
- you have a smallish bottom and bust
- you tend not to hold excess fat around your midriff
- your waistline is not clearly defined.

**You are more apple if:**
- you store body fat around your midriff rather than hips and thighs
- you are shorter in height
- you have a flattish bottom.

## WHAT'S YOUR BODY FRAME?

Here is a quick way to identify the size of your body frame – it's not scientifically proven but it will give you a rough idea. Encircle your wrist with your thumb and middle finger.

If the middle finger overlaps your thumb, chances are you are small-framed. If the middle finger and thumb touch, you have a medium-sized body frame; and if the finger and thumb do not touch you are more likely to have a larger frame.

**Remember:** for optimum health all body types need a balanced exercise programme involving a combination of cardiovascular, resistance and flexibility work. But a particular type may benefit from extra concentration on a specific component. As you continue on your weight loss journey and follow your appropriate plan, you'll see a specially designed workout for your body shape.

## HOW HORMONES AFFECT OUR BODY SHAPE

Some of us store more body fat on our hips and thighs while others tend to have long lean arms and legs but store more body fat around our midriffs. This distribution of fat is associated directly with two main hormones: lipoprotein lipase, or LPL, which encourages fat storage, and hormone-sensitive lipase, or HSL, which encourages fat to be distributed in the blood and then burnt off.
- More LPL in the belly and less HSL in the lower hip area creates an apple-like shape.
- More LPL in the hips and backs of the arms and less HSL in the upper body produces a pear-like shape.

# Pear-shaped

AIM  To streamline hips and thighs; create a visual balance between the upper and lower body.

ACTION  Emphasis on slimming the lower body while creating shape and definition in the upper body will benefit general health as well as promoting the optimum body shape change.

TARGET  Try to do these exercises 4 times a week.

## CAN OPENER AND EXTENSION

**What it does:** Streamlines outer hips and thighs and helps to lengthen and tone the muscles of whole leg.
**How many you do:** 12–16 slow repetitions on each side.

**1**  Lie on your side with your knees bent as if sitting on a chair. Keeping your feet and knees together, lift your feet off the floor. This is your start position.

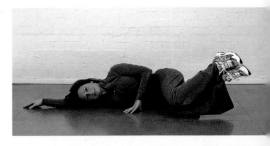

**2**  Keeping the feet together, use your outer thigh muscles to open the top knee as wide as possible and then extend the leg out to full length. Bring the leg back into the bent leg position and repeat. Turn onto the other side and repeat.

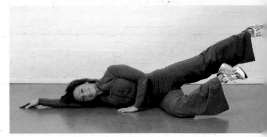

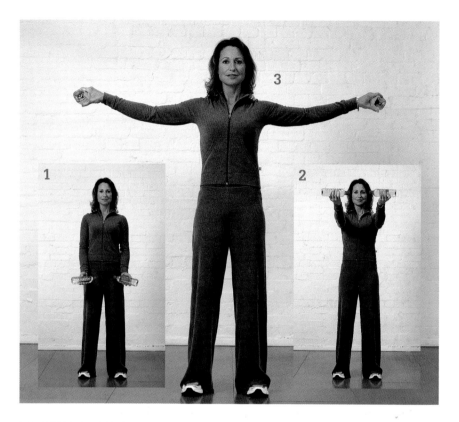

## FRONTAL RAISE AND LATERAL ARM COMBO

**What it does:** Gives shape and tone to the front of arm as well as creating and defining the shoulders.
**How many you do:** 4 counts up, 4 counts out, 8 counts down, all repeated 4 times.

**1** Stand straight with good posture, holding weights (or water bottles) in each hand, with your palms facing away from your thighs.

**2** Lift the weights slowly to eye level, to the count of 4, keeping your elbows in line with your wrists.

**3** Extend your arms out to the sides, level with your shoulders, for 4 counts and lower to the start position again on 8 counts. Repeat.

# ALL FOURS CROSS LEG COMBO

**What it does:** Targets the outer buttock area as well as lifting and firming the main buttock cheeks.

**How many you do:** 16 repetitions with each leg.

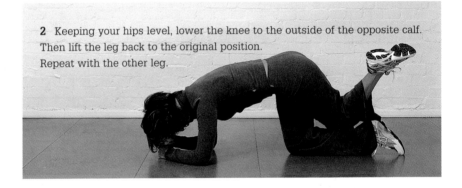

**1** Start by kneeling on all fours, then lower your forehead to rest on your hands, which should be in loose fists. Lift up one knee, with the sole of the foot facing towards the ceiling.

**2** Keeping your hips level, lower the knee to the outside of the opposite calf. Then lift the leg back to the original position.
Repeat with the other leg.

## CARDIO

Swimming can be a great all-over cardiovascular form of exercise, stimulating your heart and lungs. Breast stroke and front crawl are particularly beneficial for those with pear shapes as the strokes engage all the back muscles, helping to give tone, shape and definition. Regular swimming for 30 minutes 4 times a week will develop more shape in your deltoid shoulder muscles as well as improving your cardiovascular stamina.

# Carrot-shaped

**AIM**  To create a nipped, defined waist.

**ACTION**  There are two sets of oblique muscles which help form a trim waist; training both of these effectively will create that smaller firmer midriff. The rib cage is often expanded through stress or pregnancy, giving your torso a wider appearance. Master the rib-hip connection (see page 48) before you do any of these exercises and you will really notice a difference.

**TARGET**  Your body will benefit from doing these exercises 5 times a week.

## TOWEL OBLIQUE LIFT

**What it does:** Helps lengthen and tighten a short, thick waist.
**How many you do:** This is challenging, so build up gradually to 10 each side.

**1**  Lie on your side with a rolled-up towel under your waist. Make sure your top hip bone is directly over the lower hip bone. Extend one arm under your head, straighten your legs and pull in your tummy muscles to give support. Rest your top arm on the floor in front of you.

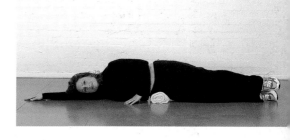

**2**  Using your waist muscles gently lift your body upwards. Try to avoid using the top hand to push you up – just use it to keep your balance. Lower your body again in a controlled manner. Do the set number of repetitions then turn onto the other side and repeat.

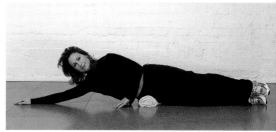

# WATER BOTTLE LIFT

**What it does:** Defines and trims the waist as it flattens the lower abdominals.
**How many you do:** Perform the whole sequence 3 times.

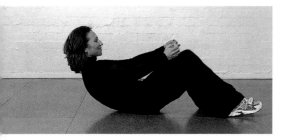

**1** Lie on your back with your knees bent and establish the rib-hip connection. Hold a water bottle in both hands. Lift your upper body off the floor.

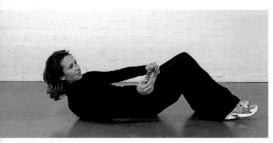

**2** Keep your shoulders relaxed and really lift up as you move obliquely across your body, extending the water bottle past the outside of your right knee.

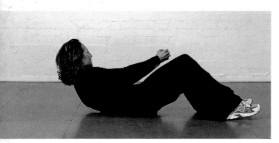

**3** Lift 4 times, stretching across to the right side, then lift the water bottle directly up over your knees 5 times before you lift 4 times across to the left side.

## CARDIO

Those with carrot shapes should focus on all-round activities. Team sports such as soccer, netball and hockey will provide a great aerobic workout as well as challenging co-ordination and speed. If you prefer to exercise alone, gym-based activities such as step aerobics and studio-based cardio classes may be more enjoyable. Aim to get a minimum of 3 structured cardio sessions in a week.

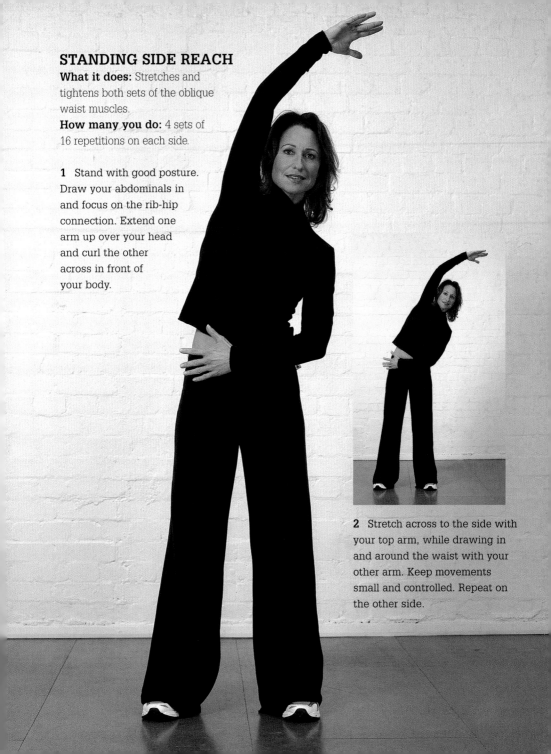

## STANDING SIDE REACH

**What it does:** Stretches and tightens both sets of the oblique waist muscles.

**How many you do:** 4 sets of 16 repetitions on each side.

**1** Stand with good posture. Draw your abdominals in and focus on the rib-hip connection. Extend one arm up over your head and curl the other across in front of your body.

**2** Stretch across to the side with your top arm, while drawing in and around the waist with your other arm. Keep movements small and controlled. Repeat on the other side.

# Red pepper-shaped

**AIM**   To firm and shape all your curves, ensuring they don't get too big.

**ACTION**   The exercises in this section target more than one muscle group at a time. This helps you get an extra calorie burn effect as well as the toning benefits your body curves need.

**TARGET**   Perform these exercises 4 times a week, along with your cardio programme.

## TRICEP DIP WITH ARM REACH

**What it does:** Streamlines whole body, tightens backs of arms and firms buttocks.
**How many you do:** 12–16 repetitions.

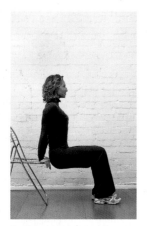 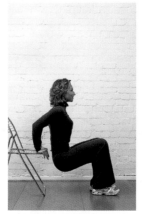 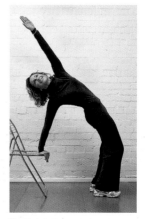

**1**  Start sitting on the edge of a chair. Rest the heels of your hands on the chair with your fingers pointing down towards the floor.

**2**  Support your weight on your hands and lower yourself down for a tricep dip, keeping your elbows pointing backwards. Don't go too low.

**3**  Straighten your arms again then press your hips forward and stretch one arm diagonally over your head.

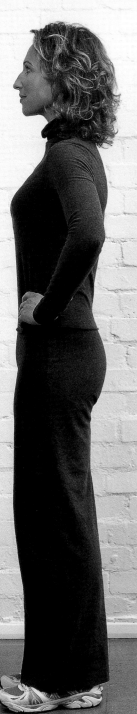

# FOUR POINT LUNGE

**What it does:** Shapes, strengthens and lengthens the thigh. A great exercise that uses virtually all the thigh muscles.

**How many you do:** 12 slow repetitions on each side.

**1** Stand on the floor (or on a low bench or bottom stair).

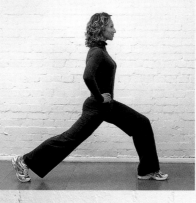

**2** Extend one leg back a large stride behind you. The front knee will be slightly bent. Lower the back knee to the floor.

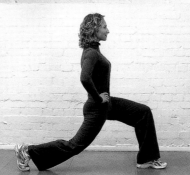

**3** Straighten your back knee then step forwards and stand up straight again, on the count of 4. Repeat on the other side, keeping your movements slow and controlled.

## TOP TIP

Check the front knee is directly over your ankle and not pushing forwards over your toe. Also check the knee is not rolling inwards. If you draw an imaginary line down your knee cap and through to your foot, it should be in line with your second toe. If you find it difficult to balance during the four point lunge, rest your hands on the back of a chair.

# MODIFIED TEASER

**What it does:** Flattens and firms whole of abdominal area.
**How many you do:** 12–16 repetitions.

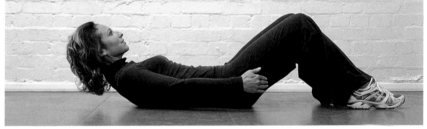

**1** Lie on your back with your knees bent and your hands on the floor by your thighs. Establish the rib-hip connection, making sure you can feel your abdominals working.

**2** Lift your upper body off the floor and place your hands on your outer thighs. Hold for a count of 4 then extend your arms over your head before returning them to the start position.

## CARDIO

Since people with red pepper shapes are prone to laying down fat, it is important that they achieve significant energy expenditure through cardiovascular exercise. Power walking and jogging are among the most accessible yet effective ways your body can burn calories. Their weight-bearing nature will also help to enhance bone density, which is important to protect against osteoporosis. As you get fitter, you can achieve variety and greater calorie expenditure by introducing intervals of skipping.

# Apple-shaped

**AIM**   To Flatten abdominals that refuse to be trained! Downsize your midriff.

**ACTION**   These effective abdominal exercises will reap dividends for both male and female apple shapes. Make sure you always establish the rib-hip connection (see page 49) before you start, to avoid straining your lower back.

**TARGET**   Do them 6 times a week. The abdominal muscle responds particularly well to being trained nearly every day – but do remember to have that rest day. Combine this with your regular cardio programme and you should soon see a difference.

## AB CURL WITH TOWEL

**What it does:** Tightens upper abdominals, especially around the rib area.
**How many you do:** 16 repetitions.

**1**  Lie on the floor with your knees bent. Place a rolled-up towel on the floor between your bottom and your feet, slightly in front of your extended fingers. Slide your feet away from your bottom until you feel your toes start to come off the floor. Establish the rib-hip connection.

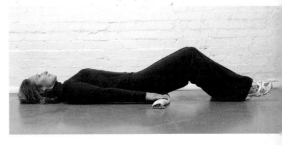

**2**  Slowly curl up from the breast bone and lift your fingers over the top of the towel to touch the floor on the other side. The emphasis should be on tucking the ribs underneath you, rather than lifting them up.

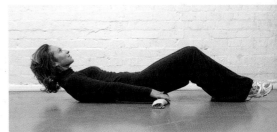

# BRIDGE WITH LEG POINT

**What it does:** Lengthens the abdominals while firming them.
**How many you do:** Complete 6 times with each leg.

**1** Lie on your back on the floor, with your spine in neutral position and knees bent. Position the legs far enough away from your bottom so you just start to feel your toes come off the floor. Pull down through your belly button, so your tummy muscles are contracted before you even start to lift.

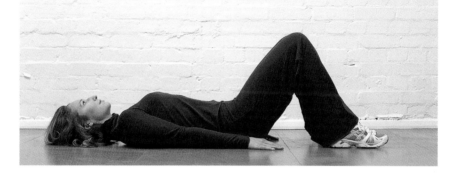

**2** Peel your back off the floor one vertebra at a time. Start slowly and use your abdominals to create the movement. Hold your abs in tight at the top of the movement and press your knees away from you, making a bridge shape.

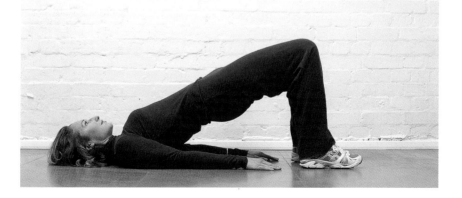

**3** Extend one leg straight outwards, keeping your knees together and your abdominals firmly contracted.

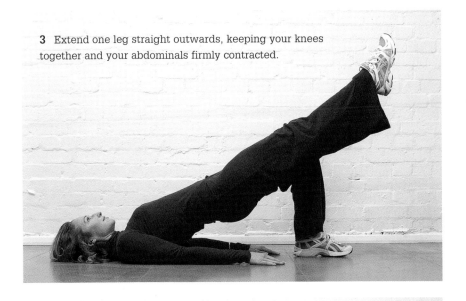

**4** Lift the leg from the hip and point the toe, then lower again. Slowly lower your upper body down to the floor, using your abdominals to control the movement.

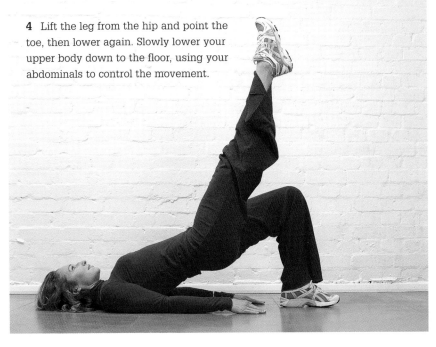

# AB CURL WITH SINGLE LEG DROP

**What it does:** Firms and flattens all the abdominals; it is
particularly effective on the difficult lower belly area.
**How many you do:** This is hard; build up to 12 repetitions,
lowering both the right and the left leg each time.

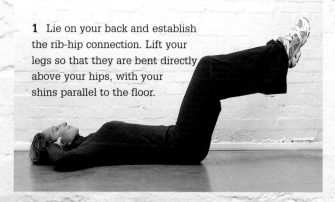

**1** Lie on your back and establish
the rib-hip connection. Lift your
legs so that they are bent directly
above your hips, with your
shins parallel to the floor.

**2** Support your head in your hands and curl your
upper body off the floor. You should feel your
abdominals working.

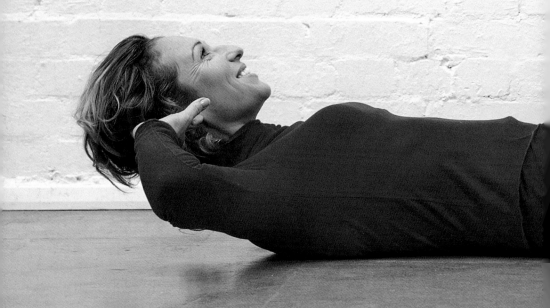

# CARDIO

Power walking and Astanga yoga are the best cardio combination for apple shapes. Power walking will provide the greater challenge, while the physically demanding nature and rotational twists of Astanga yoga will improve your body awareness in your midriff and reduce your body fat. Stress can make you lay down fat in your midriff, so use exercise to help deal with the stress in your life.

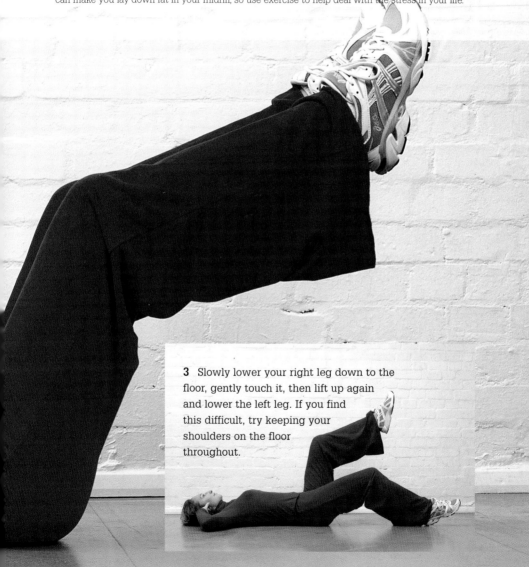

**3** Slowly lower your right leg down to the floor, gently touch it, then lift up again and lower the left leg. If you find this difficult, try keeping your shoulders on the floor throughout.

# Take action...

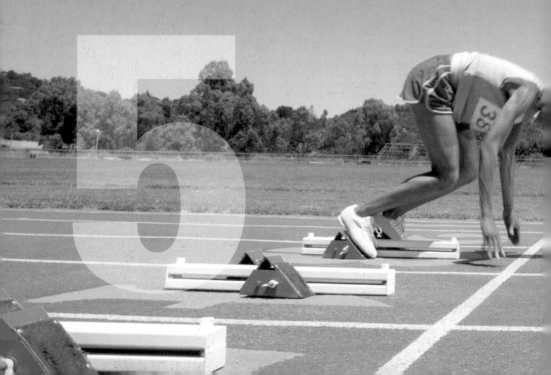

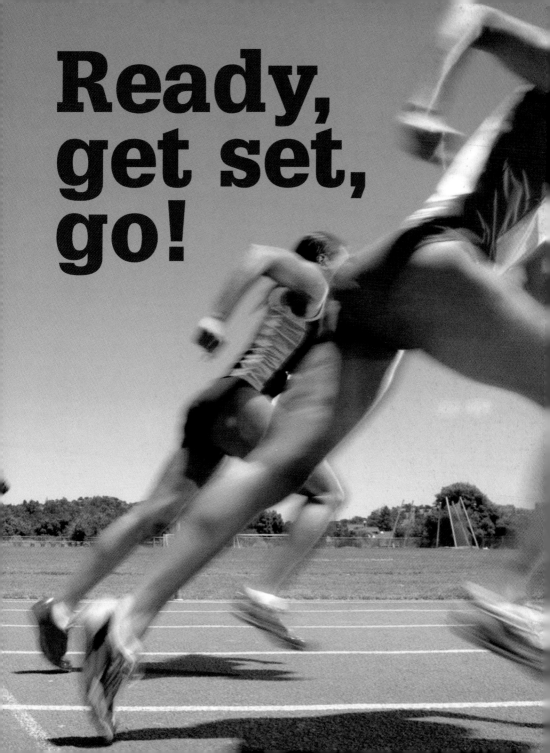

Ready,
get set,
go!

# Time to lose some weight

This is it! Here are your Action Plans. They plot out a logical, progressive and achievable way for you to reach your journey's destination. There are different plans to choose from, designed to suit your own particular weight-loss challenges and the pace at which you want to travel. This chapter is about helping you to make this happen. You'll never be more ready than you are now, so let's get going, and feel empowered! We're off!

## WHAT YOU NEED TO DO

First of all, establish which weight-loss goal is realistic for you, and choose the corresponding Action Plan. Each plan details, phase by phase, the appropriate diet and level of physical activity needed to create your required Energy Gap. The plans first of all focus on decreasing your body fat and weight with cardiovascular exercise and then introduce more specific toning exercises to shape and tone your new body. The menu plans also evolve according to your calorie needs – they will change, and this needs to be reflected in what you are eating. You may also find your eating preferences change naturally as you continue on your weight-loss journey.

## HOW THE ACTION PLANS WORK

Each Action Plan is divided into 4-week phases which have a specific theme. Each week sets out a series of achievable tasks which are progressive, helping you to realise your goals and reinforce your template of success. The exact specifics of what you eat and how you move your body I've left to you, so that you can make these action plans fit in with your life. Once your Action Plan is finished, there follows a 4-week consolidation phase to help establish your new habits and keep your weight where you want it to be.

## CHOOSING THE RIGHT ACTION PLAN FOR YOU

Remember that your aim on your weight-loss journey is to make lifestyle and dietary alterations that can be maintained for the long term, instead of changes that last just for a short period. A realistic target is to lose approximately 5–10 per cent of initial body weight after 6 months. You will not only look and feel much better but will be healthier as well. This level of weight-loss results in significant improvements in blood pressure, insulin resistance and blood cholesterol levels, and can be achieved with moderate calorie restriction and moderate physical activity.

## BEING PREPARED

Just as you would when you start out on any journey, you need to put some time aside to get organised. To get off on the right foot, you may be well advised to have a quick flick through all you have learned, just to refresh your memory.

I have designed the Action Plans so that you can achieve real success, and monitoring your progress is a significant part of this. Research has shown conclusively that the more information you monitor the better your weight loss will be, so in your Action Plans you will find a series of checklists to complete. They are designed to provide support and strengthen your template of success.

## INTRODUCE THE CARB CURFEW

Carb Curfew means no starchy carbs – bread, pasta, rice, potatoes or cereal – after 5pm. Don't panic – you won't feel as if you're about to starve, since there are still plenty of filling foods to eat. You can incorporate a whole variety of nutritious foods in your evening meal, including lean meat and fish, fruit, vegetables, pulses and dairy products, and come up with something absolutely delicious! Many of my clients consider the Carb Curfew to be the single most important tool in their weight management success and I know it can help you too. The Carb Curfew helps you control your insulin levels, which means it's easier to stabilise your energy levels – important for weight loss.

## STOPPING PORTION DISTORTION – A FEW TIPS

Weighing out the correct portion of food – 80g of meat, for example – can be a bore, so let's make things simple. To keep your meals in check, compile a handy Portion Distortion basket in your kitchen. Put in it some everyday items that are the same size as the portion of food you should be eating. Soon you'll become familiar with the sizes, so you'll be able to stop Portion Distortion wherever you are. You can still eat the foods you like, so you don't feel deprived, but you have control over what you consume and the number of calories you take in. Use the following objects to judge the portion size you should be aiming at.

| Think... | For... |
| --- | --- |
| Two dice | Nuts and cheese |
| Deck of cards | Meat and fish |
| Teaspoon | Oils and fats |
| Tennis ball | Vegetables |
| Golf ball | Uncooked rice or coucous |
| Computer mouse | Cooked portion of starchy carbs |

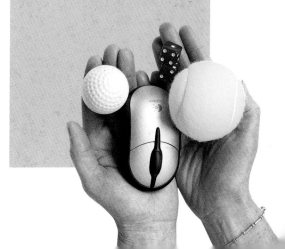

# What to do

- Note your measurements and goals in the Starting Line Form, as well as how big an Energy Gap you want to achieve.
- Select your Action Plan, based on the amount of weight you want to lose.
- Write down Menu Plans so you know exactly what you're going to eat and when.
- Make copies of the Daily Record Chart, to record each day of your weight-loss journey.
- Make copies of the Weekly Review – for identifying barriers and implementing contingency plans when necessary.

## STARTING LINE FORM

Date: _ _ _ _ _ _ _ _ _ _ _ _ _ _ _ _ _
I have selected the _ _ _ _ _ _ _ _ _ _ _ _ _
Weight Loss Action Plan.
My current weight is: _ _ _ _ _ _ _ _ _ _ _
My goal weight is: _ _ _ _ _ _ _ _ _ _ _ _
My measurements are...
Current:          Goal:
Chest _ _ _ _ _ _ _ Chest _ _ _ _ _ _ _ _ _
Waist _ _ _ _ _ _ _ _ Waist _ _ _ _ _ _ _ _
Navel _ _ _ _ _ _ _ _ Navel _ _ _ _ _ _ _ _
Hips _ _ _ _ _ _ _ _ Hips _ _ _ _ _ _ _ _ _
Thigh _ _ _ _ _ _ _ _ Thigh _ _ _ _ _ _ _ _
I am starting my Action Plan on _ _ _ _ _ _ _
My estimated finish date is _ _ _ _ _ _ _ _
I am prepared to allow 10 per cent change to my end objectives.
My current energy needs are _ _ _ _ _ _ _
My current level of physical activity is _ _
I am going to try and achieve a daily 500 / 750 / 1000 calorie Energy Gap (circle your choice)

## DAILY RECORD CHART

Day: _ _ _ _ _ _ _ _ Date: _ _ _ _ _ _ _ _ _

Breakfast: _ _ _ _ _ _ _ _ _ _ _ _ _ _ _ _ _

Lunch _ _ _ _ _ _ _ _ _ _ _ _ _ _ _ _ _ _ _

Dinner (Remember to operate Carb Curfew)

_ _ _ _ _ _ _ _ _ _ _ _ _ _ _ _ _ _ _ _ _ _

Snack 1 _ _ _ _ _ _ _ _ _ _ _ _ _ _ _ _ _

Snack 2 _ _ _ _ _ _ _ _ _ _ _ _ _ _ _ _ _

Eating checklist:
Have I achieved Carb Curfew? YES / NO
Have I drunk 2 litres of water? YES / NO
Have I watched my fat intake? YES / NO
Have I had five portions of fruit and vegetables? YES / NO

Exercise checklist:
How many steps on my pedometer have I accumulated today? _ _ _ _ _ _ _ _ _ _ _

Have I completed a Structured Exercise session today? YES / NO

## THINGS TO REMEMBER

- Although you may find it possible to lose more weight than is stipulated, it is important to preserve your lean body mass as this maintains the body's RMR, helping you to become a Fat Burner, rather than a Fat Storer.
- Some weeks you may not lose any weight at all, while the body reassesses how much you are eating and exercising – Don't be disheartened – just carry on with the plan.

# WEEKLY REVIEW

This week I completed my Structured Exercise on the following days:
Monday ▨, Tuesday ▨, Wednesday ▨
Thursday ▨, Friday ▨, Saturday ▨
Sunday ▨

This week my daily accumulated step target on my pedometer was:_ _ _ _ _ or
This week my daily accumulated physical activity was_ _ _ _ _ minutes.

This week my daily calorie intake range was
_ _ _ _ _ _ _ _ _ _ _ _ _ _ _ _ _ _ _ _ _ _ _ _ _ _

This week the barriers I bashed down were:
1._ _ _ _ _ _ _ _ _ _ _ _ _ _ _ _ _ _ _ _ _ _ _ _ _
2._ _ _ _ _ _ _ _ _ _ _ _ _ _ _ _ _ _ _ _ _ _ _ _ _
3._ _ _ _ _ _ _ _ _ _ _ _ _ _ _ _ _ _ _ _ _ _ _ _ _

The barriers that I still need to bash down are:
1._ _ _ _ _ _ _ _ _ _ _ _ _ _ _ _ _ _ _ _ _ _ _ _ _
2._ _ _ _ _ _ _ _ _ _ _ _ _ _ _ _ _ _ _ _ _ _ _ _ _
3._ _ _ _ _ _ _ _ _ _ _ _ _ _ _ _ _ _ _ _ _ _ _ _ _

My Contingency Plan is : _ _ _ _ _ _ _ _ _ _ _ _ _ _ _
_ _ _ _ _ _ _ _ _ _ _ _ _ _ _ _ _ _ _ _ _ _ _ _ _ _
_ _ _ _ _ _ _ _ _ _ _ _ _ _ _ _ _ _ _ _ _ _ _ _ _ _
_ _ _ _ _ _ _ _ _ _ _ _ _ _ _ _ _ _ _ _ _ _ _ _ _ _

I am going to put this in action on _ _ _ _ _ _ _ _ _ _

On reflection I feel I have had a:
Progressive week ▨
Maintenance week ▨
Damage limitation week ▨

My current weight is _ _ _ _ _ _ _ _ _ _ _ _ _ _ _ _ _
My goal weight is _ _ _ _ _ _ _ _ _ _ _ _ _ _ _ _ _ _

My measurements are...

| Current: | Goal: |
|---|---|
| Chest _ _ _ _ _ _ _ _ _ | Chest _ _ _ _ _ _ _ _ _ |
| Waist _ _ _ _ _ _ _ _ _ | Waist _ _ _ _ _ _ _ _ _ |
| Navel _ _ _ _ _ _ _ _ _ | Navel _ _ _ _ _ _ _ _ _ |
| Hips _ _ _ _ _ _ _ _ _ | Hips _ _ _ _ _ _ _ _ _ |
| Thigh _ _ _ _ _ _ _ _ _ | Thigh _ _ _ _ _ _ _ _ _ |

I am starting my Action Plan on _ _ _ _ _ _ _ _ _ _ _
My estimated finish date is _ _ _ _ _ _ _ _ _ _ _ _ _
I am prepared to allow 10 per cent change to my end objectives.

My current energy needs are _ _ _ _ _ _ _ _ _ _ _ _
My current level of physical activity is _ _ _ _ _ _ _

I am going to try and achieve a daily 500 / 750 / 1000 calorie Energy Gap (circle your choice)

# BE CONSISTENT

At this stage in your journey, it's time for me to remind you of a few crucial things:
- It's not how low you can take your calorie count, or how many excessive calories you can sweat off, but actually how consistent you can be with your efforts to create an Energy Gap that counts. Appreciating the importance of this right from the beginning can be a fundamental part of getting your body to work with you to lose weight and be on your winning side.

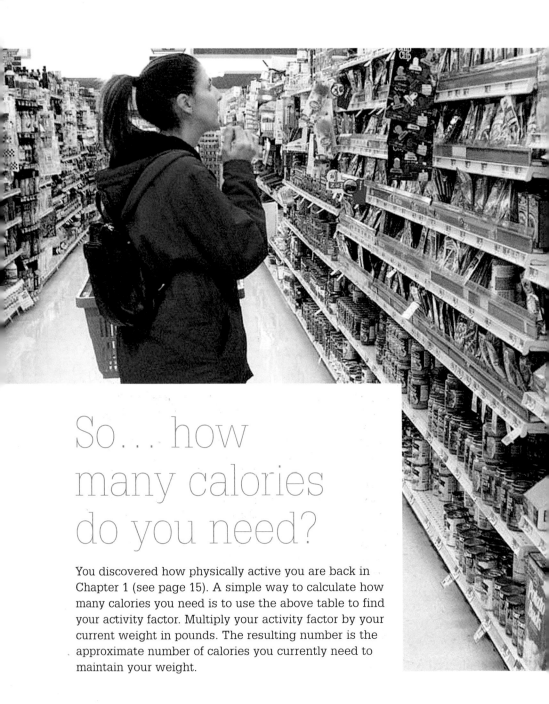

# So... how many calories do you need?

You discovered how physically active you are back in Chapter 1 (see page 15). A simple way to calculate how many calories you need is to use the above table to find your activity factor. Multiply your activity factor by your current weight in pounds. The resulting number is the approximate number of calories you currently need to maintain your weight.

## THE MATHS LOOKS LIKE THIS:

**Activity factor x weight in pounds = current energy needs.**

For example, an active woman who weighs 150lb would need 2,250 calories a day (15 x 150 = 2,250).

If you want to achieve safe, effective weight loss, reduce your result by 500, and that will give you your new target. A reduction of 1,000 calories a day is achievable, but it will be a significant decrease that will probably feel quite hard to maintain, so start with 500 calories – you can always cut back further once your new eating habits have evolved.

**Note:** Never take in fewer than 1,500 calories per day unless under medical supervision.

## GOOD EATING HABITS

**1.** Drink water, little and often, throughout the day.

**2.** Eat something in the morning – it does not have to be first thing as you jump out of bed, but eating something when you get up will replenish your blood glucose levels and fuel your brain and your body.

**3.** Eat at least 5 portions of fruit and vegetables a day – they're great as snacks and if you have at least 1 serving per meal, you'll easily make this target.

**4.** Go for colour. Check you are eating a variety of colourful fruit and vegetables – think yellow, red, green and orange.

**5.** Eat as wide a variety of foods as possible. If you can count up the number of different foods you eat on your 10 fingers, you need to add more kinds to your diet. This will help you get a greater choice of nutrients and fibre sources.

**6.** Avoid long periods without eating. This will help stabilise your blood glucose levels and make you less likely to over-eat, or grab an unhealthy snack, later.

**7.** Rate your food hunger. On a scale of 1–5 (1 = starving, 5 = stuffed). Aim to eat before you reach '1' and stop eating before you reach '5'.

**8.** Take time to eat. It sounds obvious, but it will help you eat a more balanced diet and avoid excess calorie intake. Studies show that individuals eat up to 15 per cent more calories when they are in a rush at meal times.

**9.** Chew your food. Proper chewing can aid your digestion, and has been shown to reduce symptoms of irritable bowel syndrome.

**10.** Avoid fad diets. There are no miracle foods – good health requires you to eat a variety of quality foods in moderation.

# Action Plan One

This plan is for those who want to lose around 20kg (44lb). The plan takes 28 weeks to complete and has 7 phases, each lasting 4 weeks.

**1** WEEKS 1 TO 4

**Physical activity goals:** Commit to 4 x 30-minute structured exercise sessions and a daily target of 7,000 steps, every day, by the time you complete this phase.

**Healthy eating goals:** Commit to implementing a Carb Curfew on at least 5 evenings each week.

**2** WEEKS 5 TO 8

**Physical activity goals:** Commit to 4 Structured Exercise sessions (2 x 30 minutes, 2 x 45 minutes) and build up your daily steps target to 9,000 steps, every day, by the time you complete this phase.

**Healthy eating goals:** Implement the Carb Curfew every evening in this phase, and watch out for Portion Distortion. Aim to have your portions under control by the end of this phase, and to meet your calorie target.

**3** WEEKS 9 TO 12

**Physical activity goals:** Commit to 4 x 45-minute Structured Exercise sessions and 10,000 steps a day, every day, by the time you complete this phase.

**Healthy eating goals:** Ensure calories do not dip below 1,500 a day, maintain the Carb Curfew and be sure to drink the required 2 litres of water a day.

**4** WEEKS 13 TO 16

**Physical activity goals:** Consolidate your 10,000 accumulated daily steps achievement. Aim to make this your foundation by the end of this phase. Seek out contingency routes near your home and work, so you can easily incorporate these targets. Continue with your 4 structured exercise sessions each week.

**Healthy eating goals:** Make sure you are following the healthy eating advice in Chapter 5 and maintain your Carb Curfew. Eat 5 portions of fruit and vegetables, drink 2 litres of water, keep your fat intake below 60g (2oz) each day, and eat a portion of lean protein at each meal. Plan easy-to-prepare back-up meals as part of your contingency plans.

## 5 WEEKS 17 TO 20

**Physical activity goals:** Commit to 4 x 45–60-minute Structured Exercise sessions a week. To raise your energy expenditure in each session, introduce intervals of higher intensity in 2 out of 4 of your weekly sessions. Continue your 10,000 steps a day but on non-exercise days, try to raise your daily step total to 12,000, incorporating short bouts of break-point walking pace.

**Healthy eating goals:** Introduce soups in this phase as a way of volumising your food intake while cutting calories. Remember to plan your meals for each week ahead, perhaps on a Sunday, so you are better prepared for shopping.

## 6 WEEKS 21 TO 24

**Physical activity goals:** Commit to 4 x 45-minute structured exercise sessions and 10,000 steps a day. Introduce a relaxation class as one of your sessions in Week 2 and Week 4 of this phase. Try something new, such as Astanga yoga or Pilates.

**Healthy eating goals:** Give yourself one guilt-free night a week in this phase – try some of your less healthy favourites, but watch your portion sizes. Feel confident in your newfound skills and abilities.

## 7 WEEKS 25 TO 28

**Physical activity goals:** Commit to 4 x 60-minute structured exercise sessions, using interval-training techniques on 2 out of 4 of your weekly sessions. If you have the motivation and the time, add in one extra cardio session a week, and ideally make it a longer session – try a jog, or walk a route with your family or friends that takes at least 60 minutes. Ensure you complete your daily 10,000 steps as a minimum.

**Healthy eating goals:** Implement a double Carb Curfew in Week 25 and Week 27. Choose either lunch or breakfast as your other carb-free meal. One meal a day should have carbs.

## YOUR CONSISTENCY PLAN: NOW KEEP IT OFF!

**Physical activity goals:** Commit to keeping up your 10,000 steps a day, along with brisk break-point walking and 4 structured exercise sessions each week.

**Healthy eating goals:** Keep within a calorie range of 1,500–1,800 for women, 1,600–2,000 for men, making sure you stick to all the healthy eating advice on page 84.

# Action Plan Two

This plan is for those who want to lose around 15kg (33lb). The plan takes 20 weeks to complete and has 5 phases, each lasting 4 weeks.

## 1 WEEKS 1 TO 4

**Physical activity goals:** Commit to 4 x 30-minute structured exercise sessions and a daily target of 8,000 steps, every day, by the time you complete this phase.

**Healthy eating goals:** Commit to implementing a Carb Curfew at least 5 evenings each week.

## 2 WEEKS 5 TO 8

**Physical activity goals:** Commit to 4 structured exercise sessions (3 x 30 minutes, 1 x 45 minutes) and build up your step targets to 10,000 steps a day, every day, by the time you complete this phase.

**Healthy eating goals:** Implement a Carb Curfew every evening in this phase, and watch out for portion distortion. Aim to have your portions under control by the end of this phase and to meet your calorie target.

## 3 WEEKS 9 TO 12

**Physical activity goals:** Consolidate your 10,000 accumulated daily steps achievement. Aim to make this your foundation by the end of this phase. Seek out contingency routes near your home and work, so you can easily incorporate these targets. In addition complete your 4 x 45-minute structured exercise sessions each week.

**Healthy eating goals:** Check your nutrition intake and maintain your Carb Curfew. Eat 5 portions of fruit and vegetables, drink 2 litres of water, keep fat intake below 60g (2oz) each day, and eat a portion of lean protein at each meal. Plan back-up meals as contingency plans.

## 4 WEEKS 13 TO 16

**Physical activity goals:** Commit to 4 x 45–60-minute structured exercise sessions. To raise your energy expenditure in each session, introduce intervals of higher intensity in 1 out of 4 of your weekly sessions. Continue your 10,000 steps a day. On non-exercise days, try to raise your step total to 12,000, incorporating short bouts of break-point walking.

**Healthy eating goals:** Introduce healthy soups in this phase as a way of volumising your food intake while cutting calories (for recipe ideas, see *Eat Yourself Thin* in the same series). Remember to try to plan your meals for each week ahead, perhaps on a Sunday evening, so you are organised with your shopping and better prepared.

## 5 WEEKS 17 TO 20

**Physical activity goals:** Commit to 4 x 60-minute structured exercise sessions, using interval training techniques on 2 out of 4 of your weekly sessions. If you have the motivation and the time, add in one extra cardio session a week in this phase, and ideally make it a longer session – try a jog, or walk a route with your family or friend that takes at least 60 minutes. Ensure you complete your daily 10,000 steps as a minimum.

**Healthy eating goals:** Apply a double Carb Curfew in Week 17 and Week 19. You can choose either lunch or breakfast as your other carb-free meal but one meal a day should still contain some carbs.

## YOUR CONSISTENCY PLAN: NOW KEEP IT OFF!

**Physical activity goals:** Commit to keep up your 10,000 steps a day, along with brisk break-point walking and 4 structured exercise sessions each week.

**Healthy eating goals:** Keep within a calorie range of 1,500–1,800 for women, 1,600–2,000 for men, making sure you stick to all the healthy eating advice on page 87.

# Action Plan Three

This plan is for those who want to lose around 10kg (22lb). The plan takes 12 weeks to complete and has 3 phases, each lasting 4 weeks.

## 1 WEEKS 1 TO 4

**Physical activity goals:** Commit to 4 x 40-minute structured exercise sessions a week and a target of 9,000 steps a day, every day, by the time you complete this phase.

**Healthy eating goals:** Commit to implementing a Carb Curfew at least 5 evenings each week in this phase, and try to stop Portion Distortion completely. By Week 3, introduce a mid-afternoon snack to keep your energy levels up.

## 2 WEEKS 5 TO 8

**Physical activity goals:** Commit to 4 structured exercise sessions (3 x 40 minutes, 1 x 50 minutes) and build up your steps target to 10,000 steps, every day, by the time you complete this phase. Try to introduce interval-style cardio work into your longer exercise session each week.

**Healthy eating goals:** Implement a Carb Curfew on all evening meals in this phase, and watch out for Portion Distortion. Aim to have your portion sizes under control by the end of this phase. By end of Week 7, ensure you are following all the healthy eating advice on page 87. Give yourself one guilt-free night in Week 6 and Week 8 in this phase – if you feel like it, try some of your less healthy favourites, but with sensible portion control.

## 3 WEEKS 9 TO 12

**Physical activity goals:** Commit to 4 x 60-minute structured exercise sessions, using interval-training techniques during 2 out of 4 of your weekly sessions. If you have the motivation and the time, add in one extra cardio session a week, and ideally make it a longer session – try a jog, or walk a route with your family or a friend that takes at least 60 minutes to complete. Ensure you complete your daily 10,000 steps as a basic minimum level of activity.

**Healthy eating goals:** Implement a double Carb Curfew on 5 out of 7 days in weeks 9 and 11 of this phase. You can choose either lunch or breakfast as your other carb-free meal. One meal a day should still contain carbs. If you're hungry, go for vegetable soups.

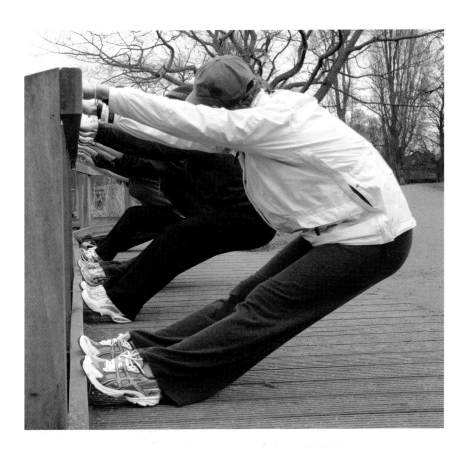

## YOUR CONSISTENCY PLAN: NOW KEEP IT OFF!

**Physical activity goals:** Commit to 10,000 steps a day, along with brisk break-point walking for at least 5 minutes and 4 structured exercise cardio sessions each week.

**Healthy eating goals:** Keep within a calorie range of 1,500–1,800 for women, 1,600–2,000 for men, making sure you stick to all the healthy eating advice on page 87 and watch for Portion Distortion.

**The 80:20 Rule:** Being consistent means you need to be good, on average, 80 per cent of the time. This allows about a 20 per cent margin for mismanagement, or slipping off the wagon and you'll still manage to lose weight and keep it off. In my experience, this rule has been enormously reassuring for my clients once they have dropped their weight.

# Action Plan Four

There are two plans for those who want to lose around 5kg (11lb). The Fast Track plan is more rigid, for when you want results quickly (5 weeks, 2 phases). The more gently paced plan takes 7 weeks and also has 2 phases.

FAST TRACK

## 1 WEEKS 1 TO 3

**Physical activity goals:** Commit to 4 x 45-minute structured exercise sessions each week, and a target of 10,000 steps a day, every day, by the time you complete this phase. Try to hit 8,000 steps every day by end of Week 2.

**Healthy eating goals:** Commit to implementing a Carb Curfew at least 5 evenings each week, and try to stop Portion Distortion completely. By Week 3 make sure you are eating a mid-afternoon snack, since it will keep your energy levels up.

## 2 WEEKS 4 TO 5

**Physical activity goals:** Commit to 4 x 60-minute structured exercise sessions, using interval-training techniques in 2 out of 4 of your weekly sessions. If you have the time, add in one extra cardio session a week in this phase, and ideally make it a longer session. Ensure you complete your daily 10,000 steps as a minimum. Revisit break-point walking, as this will ensure you are optimising your walking time and getting fitter and healthier at the same time.

**Healthy eating goals:** Implement a double Carb Curfew on 3 out of 7 days in Week 4 and in Week 5 enforce it on 4 out of 7 days. Choose either lunch or breakfast as your carb-free meal but one meal a day should contain carbs. If you're hungry, go for vegetable soups. You should feel happy with portion control and aim to have your energy-boosting breakfasts working well.

## YOUR CONSISTENCY PLAN: NOW KEEP IT OFF!

**Physical activity goals:** Commit to 10,000 steps a day, along with brisk break-point walking for at least 5 minutes each day. Add in 4 structured exercise cardio sessions each week.

**Healthy eating goals:** Keep within a calorie range of 1,500–1,800 for women, 1,600–2,000 for men, making sure you stick to all the healthy eating advice on page 87 and watch for Portion Distortion.

## 1 WEEKS 1 TO 4

**Physical activity goals:** Commit to 4 x 40-minute structured exercise sessions each week, and a daily target of 9,000 steps a day, every day, by the time you complete this phase. Try to hit 8,000 steps every day by the end of Week 3.

**Healthy eating goals:** Commit to implementing a Carb Curfew at least 6 evenings each week. Try to stop Portion Distortion completely. By Week 3 you should be implementing Carb Curfew every night. Make sure you are eating a mid-afternoon snack, since it will keep your energy levels up.

## 2 WEEKS 5 TO 7

**Physical activity goals:** Commit to 4 x 60-minute structured exercise sessions, using interval-training techniques on 2 out of 4 of your weekly sessions. If you have the motivation and the time, add in one extra cardio session a week. If you can't introduce it right from the start, make sure you fit in at least 2 extra sessions by the end of this phase, and ideally make it a longer session – try a jog, or walk a route with your family or a friend that takes at least 60 minutes. Ensure you complete your daily 10,000 steps as a minimum. Revisit break-point walking, as this will ensure you are optimising your walking time while getting fitter and healthier. Introduce the Waistband Whittler workout in 3 out of 4 of your structured workouts.

**Healthy eating goals:** Implement a double Carb Curfew on 3 out of 7 days in weeks 5 and 6, and in Week 7 enforce it on 4 out of 7 days. You can choose either lunch or breakfast as your other carb-free meal. One meal a day should contain carbs. If you're still hungry, go for vegetable soups. You should feel happy with portion control and aim to have your energy-boosting breakfasts in hand.

## YOUR CONSISTENCY PLAN: NOW KEEP IT OFF!

**Physical activity goals:** Commit to 10,000 steps a day, along with brisk break-point walking for at least 5 minutes each day, and add in 4 structured exercise cardio sessions in each week. Complete the Waistband Whittler workout on 4 out of 7 days a week.

**Healthy eating goals:** Keep within a calorie range of 1,500–1,800 for women, 1,600–2,000 for men, making sure you stick to all the healthy eating advice on page 87 and watch out for Portion Distortion. Implement a double Carb Curfew twice a week .

# Action Plan Five

There are two plans for those who want to lose around 2kg (4.5lb). The Fast Track plan is more rigid, for when you want results quickly. It takes 2 weeks and is split into 2 phases. The more gently paced plan takes 4 weeks and also has 2 phases. You don't have much weight to lose, but you will have to stick to the Action Plan you choose fairly strictly to make a difference in such a short time.

## FAST TRACK

### 1 WEEK 1

**Physical activity goals:** Build up to 10,000 steps a day, along with brisk break-point walking for at least 10 minutes each day, broken into 2 bouts of 5 minutes. Add in 4 structured exercise cardio sessions each week, making one of them a more gentle toning-style workout from the approproate Body Shape workouts. Include the Waistband Whittler workout in at least 3 sessions.

**Healthy eating goals:** Keep within a calorie range of 1,500–1,800 for women, 1,600–2,000 for men, making sure you stick to all the healthy eating advice on page 87. Watch out for Portion Distortion, and implement a double Carb Curfew on 4 of the 7 days this week. Make sure you have a good breakfast every day.

### 2 WEEK 2

**Physical activity goals:** Consolidate your 10,000 steps, along with brisk break-point walking for at least 10 minutes each day, broken into 2 bouts of 5 minutes, one in the morning and one later in the day. Add in 4 structured exercise cardio sessions each week, select your Body Shape workout and commit to this 3 times this week as part of your structured exercise session. If you've time, add in a fifth session, making one of them a more gentle, toning-style workout (such as Pilates or Astanga yoga). Make sure you include the Waistband Whittler workout on at least 3 of these sessions.

**Healthy eating goals:** Keep within a calorie range of 1,500–1,800 for women, 1,600–2,000 for men, making sure you stick to all the healthy eating advice on page 87. Watch out for Portion Distortion, and commit to a double Carb Curfew on 4 of the 7 days this week. Make sure you front-load your day by having a good breakfast.

GENTLE TRACK

# 1

## WEEKS 1 AND 2

**Physical activity goals:** Build up to 10,000 steps a day, along with brisk break-point walking for at least 5 minutes each day, broken into 2 bouts of 5 minutes by end of Week 1. Raise this to 10 minutes by the end of Week 2. Add 4 structured exercise cardio sessions in each week, making one of them a more gentle, toning-style workout designed for your body shape. Make sure you include the Waistband Whittler workout in at least 3 of these sessions each week.

**Healthy eating goals:** Keep within a calorie range of 1,500–1,800 for women, 1,600–2,000 for men, making sure you stick to all the healthy eating advice on page 87. Watch out for Portion Distortion, and commit to a double Carb Curfew on 3 of the 7 days this week. Make sure you have a good breakfast every day, front-loading your day to avoid becoming bottom-heavy with calories.

# 2

## WEEKS 3 AND 4

**Physical activity goals:** Consolidate your daily 10,000 steps with brisk break-point walking for at least 10 minutes each day, broken into 2 bouts of 5 minutes, one in the morning and one later in the day. Add in 4 structured exercise cardio sessions each week, select your Body Shape workout and commit to this three times in Week 3, and 4 times in Week 4, as part of your structured exercise session. If you've time, add a fifth session, making this one a more gentle, toning-style workout. Include the Waistband Whittler workout at least 4 days of each week.

**Healthy Eating Goals:** Keep within a calorie range of 1,500–1,800 for women, 1,600–2,000 for men, making sure you stick to the healthy eating advice on page 87. Watch out for Portion Distortion, and commit to a double Carb Curfew on 4 of the 7 days in Week 3, and on 5 of the 7 days in Week 4. Make sure you have a good breakfast every day, front-loading to avoid becoming bottom-heavy with calories.

## YOUR CONSISTENCY PLAN: NOW KEEP IT OFF!

**Physical activity goals:** You need to make sure the 10,000 daily steps achievement is the foundation of your new lifestyle. Revisit break-point walking at least twice a week to optimise your walking. Keep up the 4 structured exercise sessions each week. Ideally, if you're short of time, aim to make at least two sessions interval-style, the third session your longest workout, and your fourth session mostly toning and stretching (such as Pilates or Astanga yoga).

**Healthy eating goals:** Gradually raise your calorie intake to the level you need (see page 87). Keep your portions under control, follow the healthy eating advice and ensure you're drinking your daily 2 litres of water. Practise a double Carb Curfew twice a week to keep you on track.

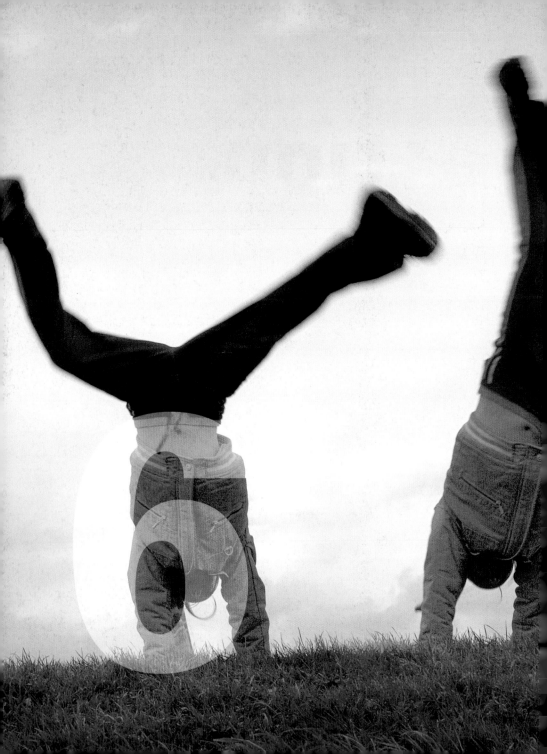

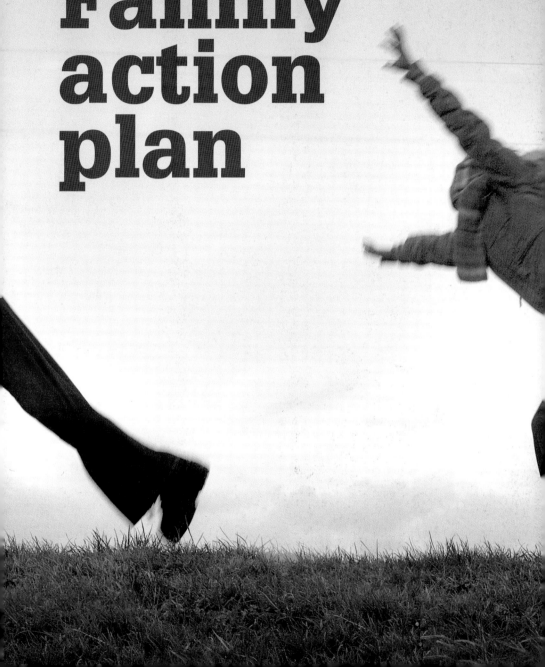

# Family action plan

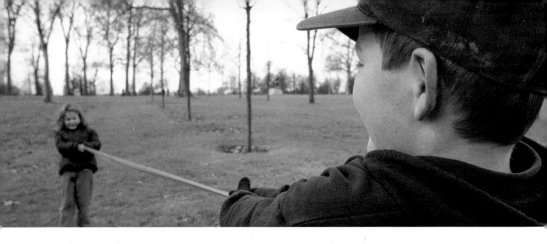

# The importance of exercise

Children are born with an innate desire to move; from speed-crawling at a young age to taking their first steps, children strive for activity and mobility. And so the fact that, as they grow older, this activity is steadily becoming replaced with sedentary video games and hours sat still in front of computers should really give us pause for thought. The food our children eat is obviously going to influence their weight, but so too is this increased inactivity as it will almost certainly lead to weight gain and obesity-related problems in their adult life. However, it is never too late to get them off the sofa and into the great outdoors!

The best and only way to ensure that your child is a healthy weight is exercise – lots of it, and on a regular basis – complemented by a healthy diet. The key thing to remember, however, is that if the whole family is involved, your child will be much more likely to stay motivated and enjoy the time spent being active. And it doesn't always have to be an organised team sport, a dance class or swimming session. Simply set aside a little time each day for physical activity, like getting up twenty minutes earlier and walking the dog with your children before school or kicking a ball around in the garden after dinner. Start small, gradually adding new activities to the routine. Even parking the car a little further away from the shops will make a difference as it means you can slot in a short walk and your kids will probably never even notice the difference!

## DITCH THE SEDENTARY ALTERNATIVES

As a time-pressured parent, juggling work, family and home life, making or taking time out to exercise becomes a significant challenge. Exercise is often perceived as a pressure rather than a pleasure, and it slips further and further down the 'To Do' list. The situation is further compounded for parents, who confuse being physically active with being mentally or geographically active. But whatever it is that is keeping you busy and making you tired, today's lifestyle is undeniably exhausting and the prospect of adding exercise to the equation may be more than daunting.

## THE INFLUENCE OF TV

Children, however, face a different challenge when it comes to physical activity. Their innate desire to move has been overshadowed by sedentary activities that we have often unthinkingly encouraged in an attempt to get a moment's peace. Children are particularly vulnerable to forms of media that require little physical involvement yet deliver strong sensory fulfilment, such as games consoles, computers and multi-channel TV.

Research has shown that outside of school, children are spending more time watching TV than any other activity other than sleeping – and the youngest children watch the most. One investigator surmised that simply decreasing a child's TV viewing by seven hours a week would reduce the risk of obesity by more than 30 per cent.

## GETTING HELP

If your child is overweight or obese, it's important that you seek expert advice before undertaking any exercise programme or change in diet. A healthy diet is, by definition, one that excludes only unhealthy foods. And an exercise programme is designed to keep kids active rather than setting fitness targets that may be impossible to reach. Don't go to extremes. The vast majority of kids will thrive on your new family lifestyle.

However, some overweight children do have a physiological problem, and your GP should be your first port of call. If you are having trouble motivating your child to change his eating habits or to incorporate a little movement into his day, most surgeries have practice nurses who can help – and your doctor may also be able to refer you to one of the growing number of 'camps' and 'clubs' for overweight kids.

To find out more yourself, you may like to read a book called How to Help Your Overweight Child (2004) by Karen Sullivan, which is full of useful advice. Weight Concern (tel. 020 7679 6636; www.weightconcern.com) has useful advice on children's self-esteem and overcoming prejudice. The Institute of Child Health (020 7242 9789; www.ich.ucl.ac.uk) has a wealth of information on all kinds of health problems in children.

## THE PARENTAL INFLUENCE

The body weight of a biological parent is the most reliable predictor of your child's adult weight. While genetics do play a part, most experts agree that our body size is dependent on more than biological predisposition. If you are overweight or obese, your child's chances of being overweight as an adult are 80 per cent greater than those of a child whose parents are of normal weight. If, on the other hand, you keep yourself in shape, then your children are six times more likely to be physically active.

## HOW MUCH EXERCISE DO CHILDREN NEED?

The Chief Medical Officer advocate 60 minutes of physical exercise for children a day, plus activities designed to improve bone health, muscle strength and flexibility, at least twice a week. However, don't get hung up on numbers as studies have shown that even 15 minutes boosts positive and alleviates negative moods. Let's get planning how your children can meet the target.

## GETTING STARTED

When it comes to taking action at home, there are several things you need to think about first of all. Before you grab your child to join you for a weekend jog across the park, bear in mind that children are not miniature adults – their physiological response to exercise is different.

Children's cardiovascular system is less like an endurance athlete and more like a sprinter. Their natural form of play is more stop-start, with short bursts of energy, so taking your children on a jog is physically more challenging for them and will make exercise seem a chore rather than something enjoyable. Stick with activities that suit their bodies.

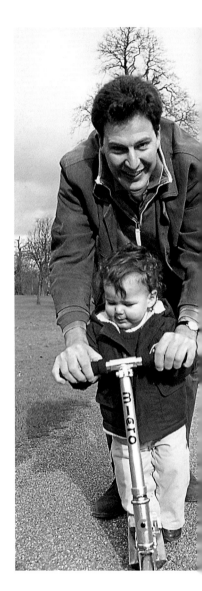

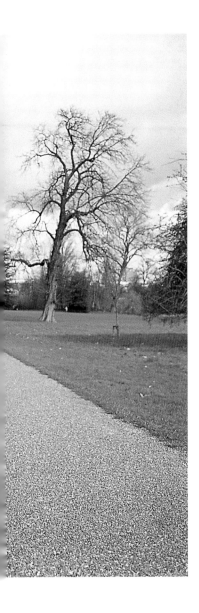

# WHY NOT TRY:

- Sprinting games and races.
- Challenges, such as keeping a ball or balloon in the air.
- Games, such as It, Stuck-In-The-Mud, or Witches and Wizards.
- Sports, such as football, baseball, rounders, cricket or even roller-blading – anything that grabs their attention and keeps them moving.
- Taking short breaks when interest flags – play on the swings or slides, or go and feed the ducks.

Aim to be physically active with them for at least an hour.

# IF YOU DON'T HAVE TIME...

The Henley Report, prepared by the American Physical Society, revealed that 85 per cent of the working population put in an atypical 9 to 5 day, with 37 per cent of parents working evenings and weekends (a figure that is, by 2020, set to double). If this is the case, as a parent you may need to think creatively about who can spend time with your children when you are unavailable.

One solution may be the grandparents, but if you don't have an extended family network nearby, it's important that you pass on your expectations to carers as well.

Consider enrolling your children in an after-school club or activity that focuses on sports or other active pursuits. Swimming lessons, Brazilian football skills classes, gymnastics, any form of dance, tennis coaching, circus skills for children, trampolining... the choices are endless. For the under-fives, you may find your local leisure centre runs a Tumble Tots class, which the little ones just love. Remember that every thing reinforces the type of behaviour you want to encourage! If they catch the exercise habit young, it will be much more likely that they'll grow up to be active – and healthy – adults.

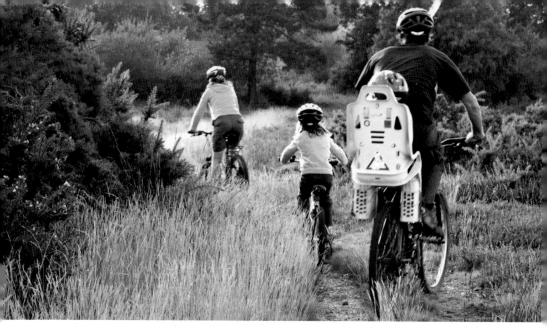

## FAMILY ACTIVITY TASK

Find pockets of time in every 24-hour period in which you can all be more physically active. First complete the 24-hour Activity Chart opposite for each child (get them to do it with you if they're old enough). You may be surprised by what you discover. Studies have revealed we commonly overestimate how physically active we are by a whopping 51 per cent. Although you may have already filled in a chart for yourself on page 15, do it again here so that your child feels that it is something you are doing together.

Next, identify the times you could add a period of at least 10 minutes of physical activity to the day. List all the family activities you plan to include.

Now, list all the sedentary activities that occupy your child, and brainstorm together to create a list of active alternatives. The purpose is not to remove all sedentary activities from your child's leisure time but instead provide a variety of both physical and non-physical activities to enjoy. And the emphasis must be on enjoyment. No child will willingly give up a Playstation session for something that's not as much fun!

Of all the activities you chose for yourself in Chapter 2, which ones can be undertaken as a family? Concentrate on those in the evenings and weekends when your child is not at school and let them join in. While it is important that your children see exercise as an integral part of your lifestyle, they are much more likely to want to be involved if your activities can easily be adjusted to include them.

## 24-HOUR ACTIVITY CHART – KIDS

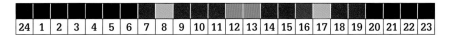

| 24 | 1 | 2 | 3 | 4 | 5 | 6 | 7 | 8 | 9 | 10 | 11 | 12 | 13 | 14 | 15 | 16 | 17 | 18 | 19 | 20 | 21 | 22 | 23 |
|----|---|---|---|---|---|---|---|---|---|----|----|----|----|----|----|----|----|----|----|----|----|----|----|

**Then colour:**

- Black time spent lying down (this includes sprawling on the sofa)
- Pink time spent on sedentary activities (in a vehicle, watching TV, playing on the computer or Playstation and even eating)
- Orange time they're on their feet (walking to and from school, for example)
- Yellow time spent doing strength training and resistance exercise (such as swimming)
- Green time spent in moderate intensity physical activity (such as brisk walking)
- Purple time spent doing vigorous exercise (such as a football match)

## 24-HOUR ACTIVITY CHART – PARENTS

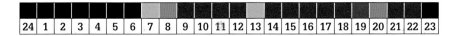

| 24 | 1 | 2 | 3 | 4 | 5 | 6 | 7 | 8 | 9 | 10 | 11 | 12 | 13 | 14 | 15 | 16 | 17 | 18 | 19 | 20 | 21 | 22 | 23 |
|----|---|---|---|---|---|---|---|---|---|----|----|----|----|----|----|----|----|----|----|----|----|----|----|

**Then colour:**

- Black time spent lying down (this includes reading in bed, lying on the sofa)
- Pink time spent on sedentary activities (at work, in a vehicle, watching TV, at a desk or computer, and even eating)
- Orange, time you're on your feet (such as doing the cooking or the housework)
- Yellow time spent doing strength or resistance work (include heavy manual lifting)
- Green time spent in moderate intensity physical activity (such as brisk walking)
- Purple time spent doing vigorous exercise (such as running)

## FAMILY FIT FACT: THIRST!

Children don't have an adult's ability to recognise thirst. In hot weather, after periods of activity, or even during a long day at school, they may be prone to dehydration, but they may mistake this for hunger and ask for food. Don't give them sweetened and fizzy drinks – they only add calories. If your child won't drink 'straight' water, try flavouring it with a little fresh orange or grape juice.

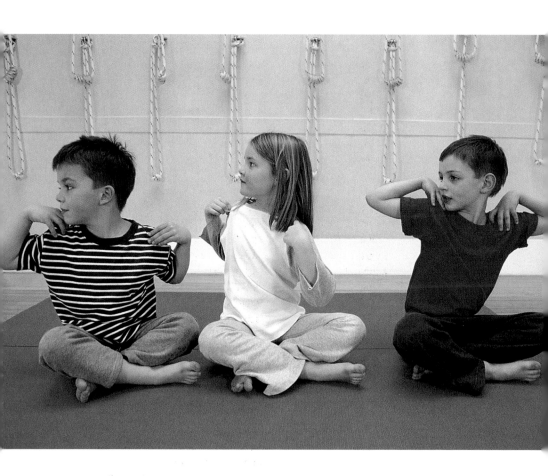

# Structured Exercise for children

Having regular structured exercise that they do every week – or even every day – gets children into the habit of planning their time around exercise, and makes it the norm, rather than just a way to lose or maintain weight. What's more, it teaches them valuable skills and, if they're ready for it, competition and team work.

## YOGA

Yoga is an effective tool you and your children can use to navigate your way through life's challenges with a little more ease: it can encourage self-acceptance, boost self-esteem, counterbalance pressure, aid relaxation, promote calmness, and improve sleep and concentration, which in turn fosters cooperation, compassion and a sense of inner fulfilment. Physically, it enhances flexibility, strength, coordination and body awareness. Once again, it's very important that you find a class that is designed for children of the right age, and supervised or taught by someone with experience.

## STRENGTH TRAINING

Strength training is safe for children over the age of about nine or 10 – it'll give them stronger muscles, bones and ligaments. In a 10-month study involving nine- and 10-year-olds, bone mineral density increased by about 6.2 per cent in those who performed both strength and aerobic exercise compared with 1.4 per cent in those who did none. It also boosts their metabolism and most importantly their self-confidence, and may help reduce the number of injuries they sustain during other physical activities by up to 50 per cent.

You'll need to join a gym or visit to your local leisure centre for this type of training, and it's important that you ensure that your child will be well-supervised, taught how to use the equipment safely, and understands how to warm up and cool down. As a rule of thumb, 20 minutes of carefully supervised and well-designed strength training, sandwiched between 10 minutes of warm-up and cool-down activities, can be undertaken two or three times a week on non-consecutive days.

## WATER EXERCISE

Most children love water – and simply messing around can be as good for them as a structured swimming session. From the gentle massaging action that helps to stimulate nerve development in the young to the soothing effects it can have on various disabilities, water is very therapeutic. Water is tactile without being invasive, so it can help tame the wild beast and embolden even the most timid. The resistance of the water provides balanced, minimal-impact exercise that safely and efficiently tones the body and improves muscular endurance and cardiovascular fitness, as well as core stability. And, not to put too fine a point on it, being able to swim could one day save your child's life!

If your child feels self-conscious in a costume, take him when your local pool is relatively quiet (or enrol him in a swimming club for overweight children), and choose a costume that fits without clinging too much.

## SPORTS AND OTHER ACTIVITIES

Despite the difficulties competition and working as a team may present for an overweight child, the skills they learn can stop them becoming a source of amusement in PE lessons at school, and can also instil a sense of pride. But make sure to choose activities that your child actually wants to try. There are all sorts to consider. What about rock-climbing, skateboarding, t'ai chi, kickboxing, dryslope skiing, or even line-dancing? As long as your child enjoys what he is doing and gets some exercise at the same time, anything goes.

Team sports can be enormously good for an overweight youngster's self-esteem. Get your child a few extra coaching sessions before they begin, in order to give them a fighting chance of holding their own (and possibly even shining). Remind children that being overweight does not mean being unskilled or unsporty. Weight just makes it all a little harder. But watch them flower in a nurturing environment, where they become part of a team and one of the 'gang'. There can, surely, be no better motivation than that!

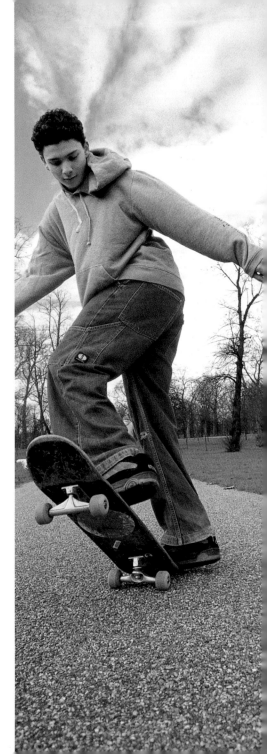

# Glossary

**Abdominals** – the group of muscles at the front of the body. Commonly referred to (though incorrectly) as tummy muscles. Aerobic capacity – refers to the body's ability to consume oxygen at cellular level and produce energy.

**Blood pressure** – the pressure exerted by the blood on the walls of the arteries, measured in millimetres of mercury by a sphygmomanometer.

**Body Mass Index** – a relative measure of body height to body weight for determining degrees of obesity.

**Break-point walking** – the way I recommend you walk – see page 38.

**Calorie** – or kilocalorie (kcal) is the amount of heat energy needed to raise the temperature of 1 kilogram of water by 1°C, commonly used as a measure of energy in food.

**Carb Curfew** – means no bread, pasta, rice, potatoes or cereal after 5pm. Carbohydrates (simple and complex) – essential nutrients that provide energy to the body. Dietary sources include sugars (simple) and grains, rice, potatoes and beans (complex). 1gm carb = 4 kcals. For more info, see page 83.

**Cardiovascular exercise (cardio)** – involves moving your body with the use of the large muscle groups. Uses oxygen as a source of energy, so it strengthens the heart, lungs and circulatory system.

**Cholesterol** – a fatty substance found in the blood and body tissues and in animal products. Essential for the production of certain hormones but its accumulation leads to narrowing of the arteries (atherosclerosis).

**Diabetes** – a disease of carbohydrate metabolism in which an absolute or relative deficiency of insulin results in an inability to metabolise carbohydrates normally.

**Energy Gap** – burning more calories through activity than you take in through your food and drink. The only way to lose weight!

**Extension** – movement at a joint bringing two parts into or toward a straight line, thereby increasing the angle of the joint. An example might be straightening the arm. It's the opposite of flexion (qv).

**Fats (saturated, polyunsaturated, monounsaturated, trans/hydrogenated)** – an essential nutrient that provides energy, energy storage and insulation to the body. 1gm fat = 9 kcals.

**Fibre** – dietary fibre is mainly derived from plant cell walls. There are two types: soluble and insoluble.

**Flexion** – movement about a joint in which the bones on either side of the joints are brought closer to each other. An example might be bending the arm. It's the opposite of extension (qv).

**Glucose** – a simple sugar; the form in which all carbohydrates are used as the body's principal energy source.

**Glycogen** – the form in which glucose is stored in the liver and muscles.

**Glycaemic Index** – classifies a food by how high and for how long it raises blood glucose levels.

**Heart-rate monitor** – consists of a chest

strap that contains electrodes that pick up the actual heart rate (not pulse rate) and transmit the signal to a digital readout on a wrist receiver.

**Hormones** – chemical messengers that are synthesised, stored in and released into the blood by endocrine glands.

**Hydration** – the amount of water in the body.

**Hypertension** – high blood pressure (above 140/90mmHg).

**Insulin** – a hormone that helps the body utilise blood glucose.

**Insulin resistance** – occurs when the normal amount of insulin secreted by the pancreas is not able to maintain normal blood glucose levels. When the body cells resist or do not respond to even high levels of insulin, glucose builds up in the blood resulting in high blood glucose or even type 2 diabetes.

**Intensity of exercise** – the physiological stress on the body during exercise. Indicates how hard the body should be working to achieve a training effect.

**Interval training** – short, high-intensity exercise periods alternated with periods of rest or less intensive active recovery. For example, a 100-yard run then a 1-minute rest, repeated eight times.

**Lactic acid** – a waste product of anaerobic energy production known to cause localised muscle fatigue.

**Metabolism** – the chemical and physiological processes in the body that provide energy for the maintenance of life.

**Neutral position** – with the lumbar spine and pelvis in the central position, not flexed, extended, tilted or rotated. Thought to be the best position for good posture.

**Nutrients (and micronutrients)** – life-sustaining substances found in food. They supply the body with energy and structural materials and regulate growth, maintenance and repair of the body's tissues.

**Obliques** – part of the abdominal muscles (qv). The obliques lie on a diagonal in the torso, forming your waist.

**Omega 3 fatty acids** – a form of fat, found mainly in oily fish and flax and pumpkin seeds.

**Pedometer** – a simple device you attach to your belt. It records each step through a sensory device registering motion at the hip. Perceived rate of exertion (PRE) – method used to regulate intensity (qv) during aerobic endurance training. Rating is recorded numerically by your own perception of how hard you are working

**Portion Distortion** – a term I use to describe over-generous serving sizes of food, for example on manufacturers' packaging.

**Probiotics** – these are commonly ingested as bacteria in live yoghurt to enhance the intestinal flora and so aid digestion.

**Resistance exercise** – involves exerting a force to enable you to move or apply tension to a weight and results in enhanced muscular strength and endurance.

**Resting metabolic rate** – the number of calories expended per unit time when you are at rest. It is measured early in the morning after an overnight fast and at least 8 hours of sleep.

**Rib-hip connection** – this helps with abdominal contraction before lifting and ensures the correct anatomical position of the spine.

**Strength training** – see resistance exercise.
**Structured exercise** – involves setting aside specific time to take exercise..
**Thermic effect of food** – is the increase in energy expenditure above the resting metabolic rate as a result of eating a meal.
**Thermic effect of exercise** – is the energy expended in physical activity.
**Weight-bearing exercise** – exercise that uses your own body weight, such as Pilates.

# Stockists

**Cassall**
Stylish active wear clothing available online at www.sportswoman.co.uk and in store at John Lewis

**Joanna Hall pedometers, books and exercise DVD's**
www.joannahall.com

**Joanna's Walk Fit, Walk Firm, Walk Off weight events, courses and spa breaks**
www.walkactive.co.uk

**Menopause matters**
an independent, clinician-led website that provides information about the menopause
www.menopausematters.co.uk

**Sweaty Betty for exercise clothing**
www.sweatybetty.com

**She Active for exercise clothing**
www.sheactive.co.uk

**Shoes**
Healthy walking shoes for work and leisure
www.lovethoseshoes.com

**Tanita Body Fat Scales**
www.tanita.com

## SMALL STEPS BIG CHANGES

Whether you want to improve your health, your fitness or to walk off your weight, a pedometer is the number one piece of equipment you need and so, in association with UK Pedometers I developed my own model, called Joanna's Small Steps Big Changes pedometer. Carrying the Gold Standard for research, this pedometer is accurate and simple to use; there are four models:

**Joanna's Elite** The calorie counting function is a major motivator to help keep you active.
**Joanna's Optimum** For those serious about their health – this multi-function pedometer will allow you, not only to measure steps and exercise time, but also your exercise intensity.
**Joanna's Duo** Essential for logging your steps and tracking your time. It's the best pedometer for those interested in fulfilling the Chief Medical Officer's recommended health targets of 30min of moderate physical activity a day.
**Joanna's Steps** An excellent introductory pedometer counting your steps with only a 1% error rate. It's a great introduction for those wanting to start monitoring their daily steps.

# Index